CALLED TO DUTY

11-14-05 —

Dear Lisa,
Hope you enjoy the book. If you could meet Kay — You'd fall instantly in love with her. She's a ray of sunshine. Anyway, I brag to her each time were together about you and our awsome friendship. Thank you for everything you do. Hope you enjoy the book — With love
Aide

CALLED TO DUTY

The Christian Nurse's Resource Book

Kay Marie Bani

11-9-05

Lisa, Ande wanted this special gift for you. May it be a blessing to you!

Yours in Christ,
Kay M. Bani

VANTAGE PRESS
New York

Scripture quotations in this book are from the King James version of the Bible.

FIRST EDITION

All rights reserved, including the right of reproduction in whole or in part in any form.

Copyright © 1998 by Kay Marie Bani

Published by Vantage Press, Inc.
516 West 34th Street, New York, New York 10001

Manufactured in the United States of America
ISBN: 0-533-12592- 8

Library of Congress Catalog Card No.: 97-91199

0 9 8 7 6 5 4 3 2

To my mothers:

Yah Yigben Massaquoi, my biological mother, a nurse midwife in Liberia, West Africa, for over thirty years, who instilled in me my love for nursing and a compassion for service to others;

and

Caroline Rotz, my spiritual mother, and a missionary to West Africa for more than twenty years, who led me to Jesus Christ as my Lord and Savior on September 11, 1979; and who encouraged me to be a Christian nurse in service for Jesus Christ.

Contents

Author's Note — ix
Acknowledgments — xi

Part One: The Mission
1. The Calling — 3
2. The Lamp — 7
3. The Role of the Christian Nurse — 11

Part Two: Things Familiar to Nursing
4. Stethoscope — 21
5. Thermometer — 27
6. Handwashing — 33
7. Nutrition — 42

Part Three: Things We Face Daily
8. Stress — 51
9. Burnout — 57
10. Depression — 61
11. Fear — 64
12. Worry — 69
13. Anger — 73
14. Pride — 79
15. Envy — 83
16. Disappointment — 87
17. Strife — 92
18. Fatigue — 100
19. The Tongue — 105
20. Gossip — 109
21. Lies — 113
22. Filthy Language — 116
23. Evaluation — 120
24. Favoritism — 125
25. Breaking In the New Person — 130
26. Hard Work/Low Pay — 135

27. Death and Dying — 142

Part Four: Things We Need More Of
28. Fruits of the Spirit — 151
29. Love — 157
30. Joy — 163
31. Compassion — 170
32. Forgiveness — 174
33. Giving — 182
34. Prayer — 188
35. Protection — 197
36. Healthy Self-Esteem — 202
37. Encouraging Other Nurses — 210
38. Taking a Stand — 219
39. Sharing Our Faith — 225
40. Tools of the Trade — 233

Part Five: Specific Devotionals
41. Newborn Nursing — 245
42. Family Care Nursing — 252
43. Nursing of the Elderly — 256
44. Emergency Room Nursing — 260
45. The Nurse in Administration — 264
46. The Nursing Educator — 269
47. Working with HIV and AIDS Patients — 273
48. The Nurse Who Is Out of a Job — 278

Bibliography — 285

Author's Note

The following people were contributors to my book:

Editor: Dolores A. Robinson

Peer Reviewers: Joseph Aviah, Ruth Kneebone, Kent Lindberg, Barbara Lyells, Dr. Susan Peck, and Elizabeth Vigil.

Typists: Dorothy Lee Carson, Mandy Mendoza, Anne Sprague, and Jean Turk.

Prayer Partners: Mr. and Mrs. Bill Berger, Pam Fountain, Laura Berry, Annette Severance, Heidi and Tim Sullivan, Will and Carol Cummings, Primus and Liz Russell, Kerry Hernandez, DeeAnn Westfall, Kathy Welsch, Marlene Ratzlaff, Kari Burmont, Mayura Yamazaki, Janet Fowler, Cindy Rogers, and Dr. Jana Wright.

Acknowledgments

The support, encouragement and prayers of many people were instrumental in the development and writing of this book.

I am particularly thankful to my son Jeffrey for his love and patience with me while I spent hours working on my manuscript, and to my sister Famatta, her husband Abraham Karva, and my niece Kay-Marie, for their love and emotional support.

I am grateful for the timely counsel, advice and prayers of my editor, peer reviewers, prayer partners and typists.

I thank Steve Heidenfelder who "saw" a book in me and encouraged me to start writing; for Karin Lilly, Anne Graham, Kathy Moore, Linda Mendoza and Marilyn Hall, who were there at the beginning, when the book was a mere skeleton; to Marilyn Chedester for her advice on using the computer, and to my sister Eunice Massaquoi for her help proofreading.

Many friends encouraged me along the way, when I doubted the value of this book or my ability to complete it. I am especially grateful to Anna Gustafson for her friendship that has meant so much to me, and to Sara Short for her love. I also thank Marva Brown, Mary Pugh, Anne Ike, Lisa Gentile, Gisa Pittel, Chris Jennison, Sharon Mann, Diane Ampe, Valerie Love, Viola Fisher, Shirley Wittman, Carol Bowen, Marie Fredricks, Jane Jaksch, Tiffany Harr, Carol Lee, and the nurses on the mother-baby units at Columbia Swedish Medical Center, for their encouragement and patience, as they listened to me gab on and on about my vision for this book.

Special thanks go to Sue Klarquist, Judy McClean, Teresa Henegan, Stephanie and David Warenski, Ruth Kneebone, Jane Hartung, Kay Cowell, and Susan "Tish" Tishendorf, for their insight, book and magazine articles, and other valuable materials used in writing this book.

I am indebted to my patients Joshua Pena, Colton Heidenfelder, Travlor and Seyler Skudneski, Emory Hoak, Abby Pulis,

Colton Northey, Emma Cox and all the other babies who have made nursing a rewarding career for me. I want to thank Pastor Billy Epperhart, the members of Trinity Christian Center, and the members of my TLC group for helping me grow in my Christian life.

Most of all, I give glory to my Lord and Savior Jesus Christ for calling me into the ministry as His ambassador to my patients and their families.

—Kay Bani, RN, MSN

CALLED TO DUTY

Part One

The Mission

Florence Nightingale is known as the founder of nursing as a profession. This section studies her life, her call to minister to the sick, her numerous contributions to nursing, and how we can emulate her courage, determination, and compassion for people in our care. It also deals with the lamp and our role as Christian nurses.

> Isaiah 6:8—Also I heard the voice of the Lord, saying, Whom shall I send, and who will go for us? Then said I, Here am I; send me.

Romans 10:15—And how shall they preach, except they be sent? As it is written, How beautiful are the feet of them that preach the gospel of peace, and bring glad tidings of good things!

1
The Calling

Perhaps no other name in nursing is more famous than that of Florence Nightingale. She brought nursing to the forefront as a career for women, and she is known as the founder of nursing as a profession. Her accomplishments in this field and many others are legendary.

Florence Nightingale was born on May 12, 1820 in Florence, Italy, the second daughter of William Edward Nightingale and Frances (Fanny) Smith. Her parents were English and wealthy. She was highly intelligent and fluent in more than five languages. She also excelled in history, philosophy, music, mathematics and art. She loved to travel, and enjoyed dancing and going to parties. She had at least two suitors who asked her hand in marriage, but she never married and had no children.

On February 7, 1837, at the tender age of 17, and even though she didn't consider herself deeply religious, Florence believed that she had heard the voice of God, telling her that she had a mission. Nine years later, she realized that her mission was nursing service. This realization changed her life forever.

Florence Nightingale was touched by all the suffering around her. Even though she was well-educated and financially well off, she chose to reach out to people who were considered "undesirables." She nursed inmates, prostitutes, the poor, and people who lived in slums, and had to cope with opposition and severe criticism from members of her family and from people in her society. They were shocked and horrified that a "genteel" woman would allow herself to associate with outcasts and people

spitals were places of filth and degradation and
a history of being drunks and living immoral
to the opposition and criticisms, Florence faced
shortages of basic necessities, poor sanitation, rat-infested facilities, and overcrowding. But none of these things could deter her from her calling.

In addition to caring for the sick, Florence Nightingale helped to bring about major changes in hospital methods in England. She established training schools for nurses, served in field hospitals during the Crimean War, and wrote several books. Kings, presidents and other dignitaries came to her for consultation. Even the President of the United States asked her advice about military hospitals during the Civil War.

She won several awards, the most notable being the Order of Merit (she was the first woman ever to receive it), but Florence shunned the limelight throughout her life. She even left specific instructions that at her death there was to be no national funeral or burial in Westminster Abbey. Her sight failed gradually and in 1901, she became completely blind. She died quietly in her sleep at noon on August 13, 1910 in London, England.

As Christian nurses, there are several lessons that we can learn from the life of Florence Nightingale. First of all, we too have a mission: to bring Christ Jesus to a world that is hurting. Jesus tells us in John 20:21b, "As my Father hath sent me, even so send I you." Christ's great commission to us and every Christian is threefold: He tells us to go teach, go preach, and go heal. As Christian nurses, we have a charge to bring a living Christ to a sick and dying world, and we have an unending mission field—hospitals, clinics, nursing homes, and doctors' offices, to name a few. All Christians are called to minister to people around them. We must minister to our colleagues, our patients, and their families. These people must see Christ in us.

Secondly, like Florence Nightingale, we have an obligation to reach out to those who are suffering, regardless of their race, creed, position in life, or the nature of their disease. Jesus Christ cares about people who are considered "undesirables." We too must care for the unwanted, the lonely and the downcast. Look around you today and see people with needs—physical, emotional and spiritual needs. We must introduce Jesus, the Great Physician, to these people.

Thirdly, also like Florence Nightingale, we must not allow anything or anyone to deter or discourage us from completing our mission. When we take a stand for Christ and Christian values, we will be opposed and criticized; we must not allow this to discourage us. The book of Hebrews, 12:1–3, urges us to keep our eyes on Jesus Christ, the Author and Perfecter of our faith. He also endured opposition and criticism, but nothing could stop or discourage Him.

Finally, we must learn to be humble. We must shun the limelight like Florence Nightingale, and give the glory to God who really deserves it. Like John the Baptist, we must be able to say, "He must increase, but I must decrease" (John 3:30). Jesus Christ must receive the glory and the honor in our service to others.

You might be thinking right now, "I am just one person, there's not much I can do to bring about change," but remember, Florence Nightingale was one woman who believed in her calling and was determined to fulfill it, so she devoted her whole life to the task at hand. If she had said, "I am just a simple woman, there's not much I can do," the great changes that came about in nursing and medicine would have been stunted. Christ can use you and me to bring about positive changes in our work place. He has called us—He will provide the necessary tools we need to carry out His great commission. Our duty is to obey Him and keep our eyes on the goal. Lives are at stake. Let us begin the task that we have been called to carry out.

Christian nurses are in a unique position to reach the thousands of people who are in great need of the healing touch of Jesus Christ, but there is a tremendous amount of work to be done. Let us start today to go about our calling, and let us do so with humility, love, and compassion. Along the way, let us be reminded by what the Apostle Paul tells us in Philippians 4:13, "I can do all things through Christ, which strengtheneth me." Paul was beaten and stoned, and he had to endure suffering and hardships, the like of which we can never imagine, yet he was sure of God's calling and purpose for his life, and that assurance drove him onward with certain conviction. Like Florence Nightingale, nothing could cause him to take his eyes off his goal. God has a purpose for our lives also, and He will enable us to fulfill it so that we can bring honor and glory to His name.

We are called to minister to others. This is our duty as Christian nurses, and we can emulate Florence Nightingale's courage, determination and compassion for people who are placed in our care.

Prayer: My Heavenly Father, help me to understand that as a Christian nurse called by You to minister to others who are hurting, I need to let people see You through me. Let me live in such a manner that Your Name will be glorified in everything I say, think, or do. Help me to know that there is a purpose for my life and that I have a ministry to bring a living Christ to a world that is dying. Give me courage, strength, and patience to do what must be done. In Your precious Name, Amen.

Thought: The true calling of a Christian is not to do extraordinary things but to do ordinary things in an extraordinary way.
—Dean Stanley

Matthew 5:14-16—Ye are the light of the world. A city that is set on an hill cannot be hid. Neither do men light a candle, and put it under a bushel, but on a candlestick; and it giveth light unto all that are in the house. Let your light so shine before men, that they may see your good works, and glorify your Father which is in heaven.

2
The Lamp

At night with her lamp in hand, Florence Nightingale made her rounds caring for the sick, giving comfort and advice, and nursing people back to health. To those she cared for and ministered to, she became known as the "Lady with the Lamp." To these people she was truly an angel of mercy because she brought them light and hope in their time of pain and despair. What a testimony!

There are several intriguing qualities of light. First, light overcomes darkness. When light enters a room, darkness is forced to flee. It is impossible for them both to exist in the same place at the same time.

Secondly, light allows us to see clearly so we can avoid pitfalls and cracks. No one understands this better than the night shift nurse who sometimes tends to her patients in the dark. Without her flashlight she would fall over patients' beds, overturn urinals, IV poles, and other equipment, and endanger the lives of her patients and herself.

Thirdly, light helps us to see the needs of others so that we can meet those needs. It allows us to see the grimace on the face of a person in pain, the tears of a person who has lost a loved one, the look of anxiety on the face of a patient awaiting the result of a lab test, and the look of joy on the faces of a man and his wife as they hold their newborn baby in their arms for the first time.

Lastly, light exposes our little "secrets"—those imperfections we think we can hide from others and from God. When there is light, we cannot pretend. People can see us as we really are.

All living things need light to grow. As the sun is the source of physical light, Jesus Christ (the Son) is our only source of spiritual light. Jesus said, "I am the light of the world: he that followeth me shall not walk in darkness, but shall have the light of life" (John 8:12).

Now, more than ever, the world needs the light that only Jesus can give. People need to know Him. In Matthew 5:14, He tells us that we also are the light of the world. Our lives are supposed to point people toward Jesus Christ, our light source.

People who seek help at health centers, hospitals, doctors' offices and clinics, need that light! The teenager who feels he has come to the end of his rope needs that light! The young man dying from AIDS needs that light! Your coworker who is going through a divorce also needs that light! When people look at you do they see that light? Does the light you produce lead people to the Word (Jesus Christ), or the world?

To be a light you must be acquainted with Jesus Christ. Do you know Him personally as your Lord and Savior? Have you accepted Him into your heart? If you haven't done so, are you willing to take that first step in faith? If so, turn to chapter 41 to learn how you can invite Christ into your life.

Ephesians 5:8–9 admonishes us that once we were darkness but now we are light in Christ Jesus, so we must live as children of light, exhibiting the fruit of the light which consists of goodness, righteousness and truth. In order to be a light to our patients, they must be able to see these qualities in us.

In Matthew 5:16, Jesus commands us, "Let your light so shine before men, that they may see your good works, and glorify your Father which is in heaven." Our purpose for being light to the world is so that people (especially those who do not know the Lord) will see the reality of the Christian faith, come to know Christ as Lord and Savior, and give the glory and honor to God.

For your light to really shine, your lamp must be clean, oiled, lit, and firmly stationed.

If a lamp is to give off its best light, it must be free of dirt, dust and soot. These things will block the light from shining through. In the same way, your light cannot shine through a heart that is full of sin, unforgiveness, hatred and envy. You must get rid of these things if you want your light to truly shine. The Bible tells us in 1 John 1:7 that the blood of Jesus Christ cleanses us from all sin. If we confess our sins to Him, the Bible tells us, "He is faithful and just to forgive us our sins, and to cleanse us from all unrighteousness" (1 John 1:9). Only He can cleanse us from all those things that block our light from the world. Let His light shine clearly through you.

A lamp must also be oiled to work effectively. Psalms 119:105 states, "Thy word is a lamp unto my feet, and a light unto my path." Your lamp must be oiled by the Word of God. You must read it daily, pray constantly, and make it part of your ministry to your patients and their families. Like the five wise virgins in the parable of the ten virgins, you must keep your lamp oiled and ready, so that when the bridegroom (Jesus) comes, you will be prepared. Oil your lamp daily with the Word of God, and your light will shine on the lives of the people you come in contact with.

Even if your lamp is cleaned and oiled, it is of no use if it isn't lit. You must light the lamp so that people can see the light. To do this, you must have a personal relationship with Jesus Christ.

Allow His light to shine through you so that people will see His attributes in your life.

Lastly, for your lamp to shine, it must be firmly fixed on the fundamental principles of Christianity. A light that is flickering or hidden doesn't give off sufficient light. In the same way, if our faith is wavering, people will not trust the power of Jesus Christ. The Bible tells us not to hide our lamp under a bushel, but to place it at the highest point where everyone can see it clearly; then people will see our good works and glorify God.

The world is in dire need of light. The darkness of sin, sickness, pain and suffering is all around us. We need to let our light shine. Someone once said, "Light is seen more clearly in darkness."

As Christian nurses, we are in a unique position to be a beacon of light that will draw people to Christ. Like Florence Nightingale, we must be the nurse with the lamp that will be a haven for patients that are hurting, sick, or dying, and for others who have been wounded by the cares of the world. Let us lift our lamps up high, so that we can say with Emma Lazarus, the Jewish immigrant who wrote the inscription that is on the Statue of Liberty:

> Give me your tired, your poor,
> your huddled masses, yearning to breathe free;
> The wretched refuse of your teeming shore.
> Send these, the homeless, tempest-tossed to me;
> I lift my lamp beside the golden door!

Today, will you lift your lamp up high, so that others can see Jesus Christ clearly and come to know Him personally?

Prayer: Lord, like a plant moves toward light, may my patients, their families, and my coworkers see Your light in me and come to know You as their Lord and Savior. Take away those things in my life that tend to block Your light from getting through, and fill me with Your goodness, righteousness and truth. Thank You for Your Word that is the lamp to my feet. May my life bring glory and honor to God. Amen.

Thought: People are like stained glass windows; they sparkle and shine when the sun is out, but when the darkness sets in, their true beauty is revealed only if there is light within.
—Elizabeth Kübler-Ross

Romans 12:6–8 Having then gifts differing according to the grace that is given to us, whether prophecy, let us prophesy according to the proportion of faith; or ministry, let us wait on our ministering: or he that teacheth, on teaching; or he that exhorteth, on exhortation: he that giveth, let him do it with simplicity; he that ruleth with diligence; he that sheweth mercy, with cheerfulness.

3
The Role of the Christian Nurse

There is no question about the importance of the role of the nurse in the health delivery system. Nurses are generally thought of as people who take care of others and who are concerned about what happens to them. Therefore, patients are usually willing to open up to them more readily than they would other health personnel. Nurses encounter patients when they are at their weakest or most vulnerable, and when they are looking for someone to trust. Lastly, the nurse is just a "call button away." These reasons and many more make the role of the nurse vital in the health delivery system.

Our responsibility as Christian nurses is to make Christ Jesus so real in our own lives that our patients, their families, and the people we work with will desire to know this Person called Christ, who can make a difference in their lives. To be a Christian nurse means to be a "Christ-like" nurse. When people look at us, they must see a living Christ.

God in His love and wisdom has given us different kinds of talents and gifts. Some people have many, others few, but we all have gifts and talents that can be used in His service. No matter how many, each of us has the ability to develop and use his talents and gifts in a manner that will bring glory to Christ. We must recognize our talents and gifts and surrender them to God to be used for His glory.

We may differ in physical abilities, intelligence and spiritual blessings. Our gifts and talents may seem so ordinary or insignificant that we may underestimate them or even fail to recognize them for what they are: spiritual blessings. A spiritual gift is simply a God-given ability that enables Christians to minister on behalf of Christ. No gift or talent is insignificant if we use it in service to others and to honor and glorify the name of our Heavenly Father.

One of these days we all will stand before God and give an account of the way we used the life He has given us. We will be judged not by the number of talents and gifts He gave us, but by our faithfulness in developing and using them in the service of others. May each of us live in such a way that He can say, "Well done, thou good and faithful servant: thou has been faithful over a few things, I will make thee ruler over many things: enter thou into the joy of thy Lord" (Matthew 25:21).

As Christians with spiritual blessings, there are numerous roles we can fill in the lives of the patients who come under our care. These roles include servant, friend, counselor, comforter, teacher and helper. These are facets to fulfilling our call to duty. Jesus Christ Himself has filled those roles in our lives at one time or another, and we must turn to the Word to understand the importance of these roles in the lives of the people we care for. The rest of the chapter will explore three of the roles we can fill in the lives of our patients.

The Role of a Servant

One of the best examples of service in the Bible can be found in John 13:4–11. In this passage, Jesus demonstrated to His disciples how to be servants, by becoming one Himself. He did so by washing their feet. In the washing of their feet, Jesus gave them an example to emulate. The disciples had been selfishly arguing about which of them would be considered the greatest in the Kingdom of Christ. In order to teach them a valuable lesson in servanthood, Jesus gave them this unforgettable illustration. He made servanthood the measure of greatness. And what better way to show this than by becoming a servant Himself? We too must be servants for our patients.

Three things stand out about foot washing. First, it is a humble service. You cannot effectively wash a person's feet unless you get on your knees at the feet of that person. Pride gets in the way of foot washing. To be effective servants for Christ, we must be humble.

Secondly, foot washing involves service to others. Reaching out to help others in need should take precedence in our service as Christian nurses.

Thirdly, foot washing blesses people. It blesses the person being served and the person doing the washing, but most importantly, it blesses God.

As Christian nurses called by God to be servants to our patients, we must be willing servants. When we look at our patients we must see people with specific needs, and we should be willing to be the instruments through which Jesus Christ can meet these needs.

What motivates a person to wash another's feet? As nurses, what motivates us to serve others? Some of us are motivated by money, appreciation, recognition or for the love of the nursing profession. As Christian nurses, our motivation should be our love for Christ. Our love for Him should make us want to please Him. This commitment to Christ makes it easy for us to reach out beyond the call of duty and serve others. Every service we render should be done to bring glory to His Name. Ephesians 6:6–7 teaches us about how to serve others, "not with eyeservice, as menpleasers; but as the servants of Christ, doing the will of God from the heart; with good will doing service, as to the Lord, and not to men."

Examples of service include little acts of kindness, a visit on your day off, simple words of encouragement and understanding, a sympathetic ear, a touch of concern, a word of appreciation or even a smile of affirmation.

Here are some practical suggestions on how we can be servants for Christ. First, we must be available to God and to our patients and their families. There must be no excuses. Jesus said, "No man, having put his hand to the plough, and looking back, is fit for the Kingdom of God" (Luke 9:62). We must get busy serving, and be willing to sacrifice our very lives to ensure the cause of Christ, and reach others for Him.

Secondly, we must be willing to do menial tasks or those jobs that others might find degrading. This will give us an excellent opportunity to learn how to be servants with humble hearts. What a way to demonstrate humility—cheerfully doing tasks that we think are beneath us!

Thirdly, we must be observant. A Christian nurse must be alert to the needs of her patients. We must look at them through the eyes of Jesus. Today people are hurting all around us, but before we can meet their needs we must first be able to assess what those needs are.

Finally, as Christian nurses we must do more than we are asked to do, and do it cheerfully, without complaining or grumbling. Volunteering to work an extra shift, or helping other nurses with their chores are good examples of practical servanthood.

In John 12:26, Jesus promises, "If any man serve me, let him follow me; and where I am, there shall also my servant be: if any man serve me, him will my Father honour." This is a promise we can rely on. We will be rewarded for our service to others. Not only will we spend eternity with our Savior, but we will be honored by God. Nothing we do for others goes unseen by God. He sees everything and He rewards us.

How can we be servants to our patients? By being an example of Christ Jesus Himself. He showed us what it meant to be a servant, and He did so with love, humility and compassion. We must follow His footsteps. Let us take up the towel and basin of water, and get to work!

The Role of a Teacher

The importance of teaching is evident in the Bible. Jesus Christ was always teaching. An important role for Christian nurses is as teachers to our patients, and the best example we have to follow is our Lord and Savior, Jesus Christ, who was the greatest Teacher of them all.

Several things stand out about the way Jesus taught people and His attitude toward teaching. His teachings were simple but profound. He used statements with such depth that many lives were changed and millions throughout the ages had to stop and think. His parables did that as well. His teachings were challenging and thought-provoking. Sometimes people didn't agree with things He said, but even this made them ponder their position. Jesus was never boring.

He taught from the Scriptures, and He taught the truth. In John 14:10, we learn that Jesus depended on God the Father, not only for the knowledge that came out of His mouth, but also for the power He displayed. This shows us that Jesus spent time studying the Word of God. As Christian nurses there are many qualities we can take from the teachings of Jesus Christ.

The nurse's role as a teacher has increased tremendously now that a greater emphasis is being placed on patients to assume self-care activities as soon as their physical state permits. Nurses regularly help patients learn to do as much as they can for themselves, so as to regain independence and function effectively in society. Because of the emphasis being placed on shorter hospital stays these days, the importance of effective teaching has become vital to good patient care.

The Christian nurse must equip herself with the Word of God if she is to meet the spiritual needs of her patients. Like Jesus, we must not only pursue and teach the truth, but we must make it exciting for our patients so that they can be eager to learn more about Jesus Christ.

We all can recall one or two teachers we consider outstanding during nursing school. Two things tend to stand out about these teachers—scholarship and enthusiasm. A great teacher must be a scholar who is constantly seeking new knowledge in her field and pursuing intellectual growth. A great teacher must also have the ability to communicate enthusiasm and excitement in order to inspire the learner.

For effective teaching there are other essential factors to keep in mind. You must establish a good nurse-patient relationship. This involves being genuinely warm, accepting or tolerant, thoughtful and patient. Your tone, feelings and attitude toward the patient and her family are very important. They must know that you really care for them. If patients sense that you are interested in their problems, they will be more stimulated and receptive to what you are teaching them.

As Christians, we must be teachers to our patients and we must strive to be the very best. We must follow in the footsteps of the greatest Teacher of them all, Jesus Christ. Like Him, we must teach the truth from the Word of God, and depend on Him for our knowledge and power.

The Role of a Friend

As Christian nurses we must also be a friend to our patients. When the word friendship is used, the picture that comes to mind is a relationship that includes such things as acceptance, love, trust, loyalty, support and encouragement. The best example of a friend is found in Christ Jesus Himself.

Love is the basis for all relationships and Jesus is the ultimate example of how to love. His love should be the standard for the type of love we should have for each other. When Jesus left heaven to come here to earth, He *knew* He was coming to die. He loved us so much, that He offered Himself to die in our place. What a wonderful expression of love! Jesus is truly our Friend.

As Christians, we too cannot be a friend unless we love the way Jesus loves. His love was self-sacrificing. Ours should be also.

In addition to love, unconditional acceptance is another characteristic of a friend. Everyone wants to be accepted, but too often we reject people who look, talk or dress differently, or who do not fit neatly into our circle of "acceptables." Accepting someone unconditionally means accepting them with their strengths and their weaknesses, and loving them. That's the type of love Jesus has for us. He loves you and me in spite of our sins, faults and shortcomings. If we want to imitate Him, we too must accept people—"warts and all," and love them. We must not allow our petty prejudices to stand in the way of the love that God expects us to have for others. We must accept people unconditionally. This does not mean that we have to condone their lifestyle or their bad habits, but we must accept them as people made in the image of God, and greatly loved by Him.

A real friend will treat you with respect and dignity. If we want to be a friend to our patients, we must not only accept them unconditionally and love them, we must also treat them with dignity and respect. When patients come to us for treatment they give up a lot of the privacy they are used to. We must remember that these people are valuable, and treat them with the respect and dignity they deserve.

There are other responsibilities to friendship. A real friend is consistent and dependable. As Walter Winchell aptly puts it, "A friend is one who walks in when others walk out." A friend is one who sticks by you through "thick and thin." To be a friend to our patients, we must be reliable. We must be the shoulder they can cry on or hold on to when they are going through rough times, and we must be the one to pat them on their backs and say, "You are doing just fine," when things are going well for them.

A friend encourages and uplifts. When our patients are lonely, isolated, discouraged, scared and confused, we must uplift them with words of support, encouragement and prayer. We must comfort them when they are hurting, cheer them on when they make progress, and accentuate the positive things we see in them. They must be able to come to us when they want a lift or when they want to feel better. That's what it means to be a friend.

Above all, a friend will make Christ real in your life. If we say we love our patients and want the best for them, we must yearn to see them forgiven, saved, and on their way to Heaven. We must introduce them to Jesus Christ. We must not only see them as people with diabetes, high blood pressure, cancer, coronary problems or AIDS; we must also see them as people with spiritual needs, dying without Jesus. People need to know Him. As Christian nurses called by God, we must tell these people about Jesus and how He saves and changes lives. We must be their friend!

All these qualities of friendship are made real through Christ Himself. If we want to be a genuine friend to our patients, we must look to Him daily to learn how to be the best. After all, we are His ambassadors to our patients.

As we serve our patients through our numerous roles, Paul cautions us again to serve the Lord, "not with eyeservice, as menpleasers; but as the servants of Christ, doing the will of God from the heart; with good will doing service, as to the Lord, and not to men" (Ephesians 6:6–7).

When we are dead and gone, all our diplomas, degrees and certifications will be meaningless. Only what's done for Christ will last.

Prayer: Lord, thank you for all the special gifts and abilities You've blessed me with. Help me to use them in service for others, and bring glory and praise to Your Name. Constantly, make me aware of the needs of my patients. Help me to be a servant, teacher and friend to the people You've entrusted to my care. Allow me to reach someone who needs to know You. As I minister today, help me to remember the greatest servant, teacher and friend—You. May my life truly emulate You. In Your Precious Name. Amen.

Thoughts: The purpose of life is to serve and to show compassion and the will to help others. Only then have we ourselves become true human beings.
—Albert Schweitzer

Do what you can, with what you have, where you are.
—Theodore Roosevelt

Part Two

Things Familiar to Nursing

In this section, familiar instruments and terms pertaining to nursing are studied, and analogies are drawn between these and valuable attributes for Christian living.

> Hebrews 4:12—For the word of God is quick, and powerful, and sharper than any two-edged sword, piercing even to the dividing asunder of soul and spirit, and of the joints and marrow, and is a discerner of the thoughts and intents of the heart.

Ezekiel 36:26—A new heart also will I give you, and a new spirit will I put within you: and I will take away the stony heart out of your flesh, and I will give you an heart of flesh.

4
Stethoscope

In 1819, French Physician Rene Laënnec (1781–1826) introduced the stethoscope to medicine. The stethoscope is an instrument which assists in the assessment of the condition of the heart, lungs and abdomen. It is used to determine how the heart is functioning, and to diagnose problems.

Our society has increasingly become a "heart-conscious" society. Experts in books and on television warn us daily about salt intake, cholesterol levels, fat intake, and the dangers of smoking. Tips are given on how to reduce stress and prolong life, and we are encouraged constantly to walk, run, or do other types of exercise—all for one goal—to keep the heart fit.

There is no question about the importance of the heart to the body. The heart is the center of our physical being. Without it, the physical body ceases to function. Fitness of the heart is, therefore, critical.

The Bible is also concerned about the fitness of the heart, but unlike human physicians, God doesn't need stethoscopes to listen to our hearts and to diagnose our problems. The Bible tells us He sees and knows everything about us (2 Chronicles 6:30). Nothing is hidden from Him. He knows our most secret thoughts (Psalm 44:21). Hebrews 4:13 tells us that everything is bare before God, so we cannot deceive Him, no matter how hard we try! God created the heart. He knows every artery, vein and chamber, and if something is wrong with the heart, He alone can fix it. His treatment is complete. He fixes it physically, emotionally, and most importantly, spiritually.

God recognizes heartaches, broken hearts, faint hearts, hardened hearts, evil and perverse hearts, anxious hearts, and wounded hearts. He also understands symptoms of spiritual heart disease, such as deceitfulness, hatred, prejudice, hypocrisy, and spiritual struggle. All these symptoms are examples of spiritual "fatty deposits" that clog our spiritual arteries. Ezekiel 36:26 tells us that God can give us a brand-new heart, a transplant, when our old, sick, unrepentant and unforgiving heart is removed and replaced with a pure, loving, open and whole heart which is receptive to God and His Word.

The first physical heart transplant was performed by Christiaan Barnard at Groote Schuur Hospital in Cape Town, South Africa, on December 3, 1967. Long before this physical transplant, however, God spoke in the Old Testament about the need for a change of heart.

There are some similarities between physical and spiritual heart transplants. First, in both cases the patient has to have faith in the physician. For the spiritual transplant, you must believe that God is able to do this transplant. Secondly, in both cases, you must give your consent for the transplant to take place. Just like the consent form that has to be signed before the physical surgery is performed, you must give your consent to God before the spiritual surgery can take place. God does not force you. You must have a desire for it. Your will and choice come into play.

Thirdly, in both cases someone has to die in order for the transplant to take place. In the physical transplant, the frail, brain-dead donor has to die if his heart is to be used. In the spiritual transplant, Jesus Christ, the King and Son of God, has already died so that we can get the new heart.

A fourth similarity is that both transplants need pre-op orders. The orders for the physical transplant might include lab work, special tests, type and cross-match, and fasting. The spiritual transplant also has pre-op orders. It involves the confession of our sins, a broken and contrite spirit, and confession of our need for Christ Jesus.

Finally, in both transplants, we require maintenance and periodic checkups after surgery. In the physical transplant, the patient needs anti-rejection medications, teaching, and rehabilitation. In the spiritual transplant, our new heart requires the maintenance of daily Bible study and prayer, and fellowship with other Christians. The periodic checkups involve allowing God (the Physician) to constantly inspect the new heart to maintain its fitness. It also involves allowing the Holy Spirit to teach and to remind us daily of the types of exercise we need.

There are major differences between the transplants. The physical transplant is costly, painful, and time-consuming, but the spiritual transplant is free of charge, painless, and instant. The physical transplant is temporary, but the spiritual transplant is for eternity. When God does His transplant, He gives us a brand-new heart, not one that has been recycled. His transplant brings about a change in our lives, our relationships, our work, and our play; and God gives us a bonus—a new spirit that will teach us how to live to the fullest. This new spirit empowers, energizes and strengthens us.

Finally, when He does His transplant, God removes the stony, evil and broken heart and replaces it with a heart that is whole, pure and steadfast. Let's look at the heart before and after the spiritual transplant.

Before the Spiritual Transplant:

1. Heavy Heart: (Proverbs 14:13) The heart is the focal point of the emotions and can therefore be weighed down with worry, fear, stress, depression, guilt, loneliness, unconfessed sins, and lack of forgiveness. All these things drain our energy and make us weak and tired.
2. Wounded and Broken Heart: (Psalm 147:3) Sometimes this is caused by disappointments in people and circumstances, lost loves, lost opportunities, and a loss of faith.
3. Fearful Heart: (John 14:27) Fear causes us to lose sight of our goal of reaching others for Christ. It also causes us to doubt the power of God in our lives.
4. Hardened Heart: (Hebrews 3:8) Like atherosclerosis,

fatty deposits of unconfessed sins clog and desensitize the heart and make it useless for God's service. The hardened heart also refuses to forgive others.
5. <u>Proud Heart:</u> (Proverbs 28:25) This makes a person think he is better than or superior to other people. It makes us think we are self-sufficient, without dependence on the strength of God.
6. <u>Evil and Wicked Heart:</u> It appears that Satan himself has taken up residence here. This heart partakes in evil and wicked acts that go against everything Jesus Christ stands for.
7. <u>Perverse Heart:</u> (Proverbs 12:8) A perverse heart will do immoral and perverse things that harm the body and hurt God and other people.
8. <u>Sick Heart:</u> (Proverbs 13:12) This is a heart diseased by hatred, prejudice, and an unforgiving spirit.
9. <u>Calloused Heart:</u> (Isaiah 6:10) Here is a heart that is desensitized and numbed, and appears blinded to the needs of others.
10. <u>Angry Heart:</u> (2 Corinthians 2:4) It is a heart that acts in such a way as to ruin our testimony.
11. <u>Deceitful Heart:</u> (Jeremiah 17:9) A heart that specializes in lies, gossip, slander, and "putting others down," its best suit is the mask of pretense.
12. <u>Troubled Heart:</u> (John 14:1) A heart that forgets our Father is the King Who owns everything, this heart would rather sit and worry instead of taking steps in faith. This heart is also weighed down by the cares of this world.

After the Spiritual Transplant the heart becomes:

1. <u>A New Heart:</u> (Ezekiel 36:26) A brand-new heart that brings about major changes in our lives.
2. <u>Whole Heart:</u> (Psalm 119:145) A self-sacrificing heart that has one goal—serving God and others.
3. <u>Undivided Heart:</u> (Psalm 86:11) A consistent and sta-

ble heart that takes a stand for what it believes in, even if it means being politically incorrect.

4. Secure Heart: (Psalm 112:8) A heart that is secure, confident and established in the power and strength of the Holy Spirit.
5. Sound Heart: (Proverbs 14:30) A heart that is grounded in the Word of God and can back up its testimony with truth.
6. Pure Heart: (Proverbs 22:11) A heart that is washed daily by the Word of God.
7. Gentle and Humble Heart: (Matthew 11:29) A heart that is Spirit-filled and bearing fruit.
8. Clean Heart: (Psalm 51:10) A heart that doesn't harbor grudges, and one that refuses to indulge in gossip, lies, filthy language, immoral thoughts and other attitudes that soil a person.
9. Wise and Discerning Heart: (Proverbs 10:8, 1 Kings 3:12) A spirit-filled heart that can tell the difference between the truth of Jesus Christ and the lies of the Devil.
10. Steadfast Heart: (Psalm 108:1) A heart fixed on Jesus Christ, and which takes a stand that brings glory to Him. A heart that doesn't waver.
11. Upright Heart: (Psalm 125:4) A heart that believes in Christian values and actually lives by these values.
12. Glad Heart: (Acts 2:46) A heart that has contagious joy, happiness, and peace which the world can never understand.
13. Responsive Heart: (2 Kings 22:19) A heart that has a teachable spirit, is opened, and is allowing the Holy Spirit to work. A humble and tender heart that is eager to know Jesus Christ more and more each day.

As nurses we know how important the heart is to the body. When something goes wrong with the heart, the body is in lots of trouble.

In the same way, as Christians we know how important it is to have a clean, sincere and steadfast heart, one that God can use in His service. When we allow God to give us a new heart, it makes it easier to serve Him as we should, and it sustains us for our service to others.

Do you have a heavy, sick or wounded heart today? Is your heart calloused from deceit, pride, unconfessed sins, and a lack of forgiveness? Is your heart aching or broken? Or is your heart so desensitized and numb that you don't even care about your spiritual life or the spiritual life of those in your care? If the answer to any of these questions is yes, you need a spiritual heart transplant. Why don't you allow the Great Physician to use His heavenly stethoscope to diagnose your problem and then allow Him to give you a new, upright, pure, sound, secure and gentle heart.

Prayer: My Heavenly Father, today I pray along with the psalmist: "Create in me a clean heart, O God; and renew a right spirit within me." Transform my heart so that my life can be a testimony for You, and fill my heart that I may care for others with the love and compassion of Your Son, Jesus Christ. Amen.

Thought: A physical healing will affect an individual for as long as he lives physically, but transformation of the heart lasts forever.

—Ted Roberts

John 14:26—But the Comforter, which is the Holy Ghost, whom the Father will send in my name, he shall teach you all things, and bring all things to your remembrance, whatsoever I have said unto you.

5
Thermometer

The Italian astronomer Galileo is sometimes given credit for inventing the first thermometer. Others, like Santorio (1561–1636) and Huygens (1629–1695) also experimented with thermometric instruments, but the mercury thermometer used widely today was designed in 1714 by German physicist Gabriel D. Fahrenheit. The common glass thermometer has two parts: the stem and the bulb. The bulb holds mercury, a metal which expands when exposed to heat. As the mercury expands, it moves into the calibrated stem.

An elevated temperature known as pyrexia, or fever, is a common symptom of illness. Fever is a form of warning that lets the nurse or physician know that something is not right somewhere in the body. A temperature below normal (hypothermia) is very dangerous, especially in infants. Interestingly, both fever and hypothermia can be of benefit as well as danger. Evidence indicates that fever can actually aid the body in fighting illness by destroying bacteria and mobilizing the body's defenses to fight the disease. Hypothermia causes body functions to slow down, thereby decreasing the demand for oxygen. This reaction can act to save people submerged in icy water, allowing them to be revived even after several minutes in the water.

Both fever and hypothermia are symptoms that warn us of trouble in the body. As Christians, we also have a device that lets us know when something is spiritually wrong within us. It is called the Holy Spirit, and He makes us aware of the problem and provides a solution so we can become effective, productive, and healthy witnesses for Jesus Christ.

The Holy Spirit is the third Person of the Trinity, along with the Father and the Son. As such, the Holy Spirit possesses all the attributes of personality: Mind (Romans 8:27); Knowledge (1 Corinthians 2:10–11); and Will (1 Corinthians 12:11). The Holy Spirit is equal in every way to the Father and the Son. Before Jesus went to the cross, He prepared His disciples by telling them about the Comforter, Helper and Counselor who would come after He had gone. The Holy Spirit would come to do for them what Jesus had been to them (John 14:16).

Jesus gave His disciples the assurance that He would not leave them comfortless to face the world alone. The Holy Spirit would be with them every day and forever, even to the end of time.

Jesus was thirty years old when the Holy Spirit came upon Him. Before then, not much is known about His ministry. "No mighty works are mentioned until after the Holy Spirit came upon Him. Only then did Jesus dare to embark on his public ministry."[1] It was then that Jesus attempted to do mighty works of teaching and healing. Three years later, on the way to the cross, He commanded His disciples to wait in Jerusalem until they too had experienced the power of the Holy Spirit, which would enable them to preach, teach, and witness to others (Acts 1:8). "Only the Holy Spirit could give them the ability to communicate truth to other people; could supply them with in-depth perception into the needs of others; could give them a message; convict of sin; heal; administer the infant church—in short, equip them for service."[2]

Before they became Spirit-filled, the disciples were just ordinary Christians. Then, something happened, something wonderful that changed their lives forever. The Holy Spirit came upon them, and these Spirit-filled men began to be used mightily by God. Peter, who might have been described as a timid, fickle liar (remember that he denied Jesus Christ three times), became known as the bold and brave Peter of Pentecost who wasn't afraid to preach about Jesus Christ to people he knew were dangerous to him. In fact, except for John (who died in exile on the

Isle of Patmos), all the disciples died a martyr's death. When they became Spirit-filled, they became brave, courageous, and victorious. Fear and doubt melted away and, to them, nothing was more important than telling the world about Jesus Christ and His saving grace.

Have you ever asked yourself why some Christian caregivers stand out in their workplace? They are genuine, confident, and powerful witnesses for Jesus Christ. They are not ashamed of their love for Jesus Christ, and they are willing to go the extra mile to let the world know that He is in charge of their lives. For them, it is more important to be right with God than to be considered "politically correct."

These people seem to have that special boldness, power, and radiance that makes people want to stop and listen to them. They are energetic and vibrant, and always eager to talk of Jesus Christ and about what He has done in their lives. They study the Word of God daily, and memorize verses to use when witnessing to others. It is very easy for them to lead others to Christ. They can do these things that we find difficult because they are Spirit-filled Christians. They have allowed the Holy Spirit expression in their lives, thus they have that special boldness and radiance that sets them apart from other caregivers who say they are Christians.

It is very important to understand the Spirit-filled life. When you are born again, the Holy Spirit comes to live within you (Romans 8:9 and 14) but, as David Hocking puts it, "You may have the Holy Spirit, but that doesn't mean the Holy Spirit has you." We must be Spirit-filled if the Holy Spirit is to be made manifest in us as Christian caregivers. We need the energy flow of the Holy Spirit to reach people who are in desperate need of Christ Jesus. We need to be filled to overflowing so that our joy and radiance can touch our patients, their families, and those with whom we work.

Many of us are not Spirit-filled because we don't *allow* the Spirit in. "Believers can often ignore the ministry and work of the Holy Spirit. They hear of wild and fanciful interpretations of how the Holy Spirit works, and they want nothing to do with this. But the Holy Spirit is God! He lives inside the body of every believer (1 Corinthians 6:19) and He is our greatest resource, along with the Bible, for living the Christian life. We cannot afford to neglect or ignore His presence and power."[3] We must not reject, grieve, or quench the Holy Spirit.

Rejecting the Spirit

We hinder the Holy Spirit by rejecting the laws and principles of God. The dictionary definition of rejecting is "to refuse to take, agree to, use, or believe in something." When we refuse to believe in the power of the Holy Spirit, we reject the laws God has laid down for us. This occurs often in the area of sexual purity. For instance, I know a fellow who was once "on fire" for Christ, but because of sexual immorality he can no longer lead a victorious life. Prior to his sexual acting out, he could talk about the saving grace of Jesus Christ, and could lead people to Him easily. Now, he cannot even say the name of Jesus. Before, he could spend hours telling others about how Christ Jesus can change lives. Now, he can only sit and feel sorry for himself. He still has the Holy Spirit living in him, but he has squandered his joy, confidence, energy, and vibrancy on his sexual immorality. He has rejected the power of the Holy Spirit.

Sexual purity is one of the laws laid down by God. When we break that law, we reject the Holy Spirit. It is wrong to have sexual relationships outside the marital bond. Until we practice God's laws, the power of the Holy Spirit cannot be manifested in our lives. Galatians 5:16 tells us to walk in the Spirit, so as not to fulfill the lust of the flesh. It is impossible to walk in the Spirit and continue to disobey God's laws.

Grieving the Spirit

Ephesians 4:30 tells us, "And grieve not the Holy Spirit of God, whereby ye are sealed unto the day of redemption." We grieve the Holy Spirit by our words, attitudes, and reactions. The way we treat people seriously affects the Holy Spirit Who lives inside of us. Ephesians 4:25–31 lists those things that grieve the Holy Spirit. They are lying, sinning because of anger, stealing, corrupt communication, bitterness, wrath, clamor, evil speaking, and malice. When we do these things, we are breaking the heart of the Holy Spirit who lives inside us, and this hinders the manifestation of His power in our lives.

Quenching the Spirit

To quench means to extinguish, as in fire with water. The Holy Spirit is like a fire ignited within us, and we can quench that flame by our words and actions. When we allow disappointments, lack of forgiveness, strife, unresolved anger, and wrongdoing to rob us of the joy we should be sharing in Christ, we quench the Holy Spirit. When we don't confess hidden sins or give thanks to God for all He has done for us, we quench the Holy Spirit. The power of the Holy Spirit cannot be seen in our lives when we allow things into our lives which cause us to lose our joy and peace, or cause us to forget to glorify God the way we should. When we are tempted to let resentment and bitterness set in and take hold of us after we've been unfairly treated, especially in the workplace, this quenches the work of the Holy Spirit in our lives.

The Holy Spirit longs to strengthen, energize, and empower us, but that cannot happen when we pour water over His fire in us. The Holy Spirit longs to bring radiance, boldness, joy, and courage to believers in Christ and fit us for service to others. We need this power to reach our patients, their families, and our co-workers.

Just as fever protects the body by destroying bacteria and mobilizing the body's defenses to fight disease, and as hypothermia slows down body functions and decreases the demand for oxygen, the Holy Spirit longs to protect us and help us to control our sinful desires. The Holy Spirit teaches us to pray, guides our actions, and makes us understand and remember God's truth. We are given a "fever" of love, joy, goodness and faith to be witnesses for Christ Jesus. The Holy Spirit also gives us the "hypothermia" of meekness, gentleness, patience, temperance, and self-control, in order to help us in our ministry to others. If we want to live a victorious life, let us stop hindering the work of the Holy Spirit in our lives, and instead let that power make us dynamic Christian caregivers. Let us allow the Holy Spirit's power into our lives, and let us do so today.

Prayer: Holy Spirit, thank You for coming into my heart to live, and for being my Helper, Comforter, Companion and Friend. Fill me to excess, so that Your Power may flow through me and touch the lives of all who come in contact with me today. Give me the courage and boldness to reach even the most difficult people. In the precious name of Jesus Christ. Amen.

Thought: The great purpose in the filling of the Holy Spirit is power for service. The best and most-used Christians known to me have been men who have testified to a deeper experience of the filling of the Holy Spirit.

—J. Edwin Orr

Notes

1. Catherine Marshall, *The Helper: He Will Meet Your Needs* (Old Tappan, NJ: Fleming H. Revell Company, 1978), p. 25.
2. Ibid., p 26.
3. David Hocking, *The Dynamic Difference* (Eugene, OR: Harvest House Publishers), p. 149.

Psalm 51:7—Purge me with hyssop, and I shall be clean: Wash me, and I shall be whiter than snow.

6
Handwashing

In the middle of the 19th century, Hungarian physician Ignaz Philipp Semmelweis observed that many patients died after they had been examined and cared for by medical students and doctors who had come directly from autopsies, to the maternity ward.

As he continued to investigate, he concluded that the doctors and students who came directly from the dissecting room to the maternity ward carried infections from diseased patients, to the healthy mothers. He therefore suggested that the doctors and students wash their hands in a special chlorine solution after each autopsy. This measure promptly reduced the mortality rate from 18.27 to 1.25 percent.

Still later, he encouraged his students to wash their hands after examining each living patient, and the mortality rate dropped even further.

Despite this astonishing discovery, his superior and his colleagues were very critical of him and refused to accept his ideas. This controversy eventually took its toll. He lost his job, and in 1865, he suffered a breakdown and was taken to a mental institution, where he died without being recognized for the great achievement he had brought to medicine.

His doctrine was eventually accepted by medical science and is still practiced faithfully to this day.

There is no question that the single most important factor in the prevention and spread of infection in the hospital is good handwashing technique. Nurses should wash their hands when they come on duty, before and after contact with patients, before and after procedures, any time hands become soiled, when duty is complete, and before leaving the workplace.

Good handwashing prevents the spread of infection between the caregiver and the patient, and from one patient to another. As the saying goes, "An ounce of prevention is better than a pound of cure." It costs far less to wash our hands than to treat a patient for an infection caused by negligence in nursing care. Good handwashing not only helps the patients, it protects the caregivers from infection, as well.

Exodus 30:20–21 teaches that before entering the tabernacle, it was mandatory for the priest to wash his hands and feet at the laver, cleansing himself from defilement. If he didn't do this, the Bible states, he would die.

We, as Christians who are referred to as a royal priesthood (1 Peter 2:9), need cleansing daily by the Word of God. If you and I fail to receive this cleansing, we begin to die spiritually, and become useless to ourselves and to God in His service to mankind. Ephesians 5:26 reveals, "that he might sanctify and cleanse it with the washing of water by the word." It is indeed very important that we study and meditate on the Word of God. Like the handwashing we do to prevent the spread of infection in the hospital, we need a continuous and daily washing by the Word of God so we do not infect our testimonies and risk spiritual death.

I don't know about you, but when I am not going daily to the Word of God, I begin to feel spiritually sick. I say things I shouldn't say and do things that don't bring glory to Jesus Christ. It becomes easier to disobey God and to allow disappointment and discouragement to cloud my life. I find it difficult to pray or to find joy in the things that lift up Jesus Christ. There is no question that many of the hardships and difficulties we experience as Christians can be traced to a lack of daily Bible study and prayer time.

The Word of God (the Bible) is considered the world's number one best-seller, but it is also suggested that it may be the least read best-seller in the world! We can agree that it is the most important book in the world, but how many of us really spend time reading and studying the Bible? We take great pride in possessing one, and in America most homes have two or three copies. There are those who carry the Bible around with them to "make a statement." Some people have Bibles with expensive bindings, or very large Bibles. Some use the Bible for decoration in their homes, or to impress visitors. Sometimes the Bible serves as a flower press, or storage for photos, but far too many are dust collectors.

Do you study it? Meditate on it? Memorize parts of it daily? Most importantly, do you live by it?

Many people find the Bible difficult to understand. There are two major reasons why people find it hard to read the Bible every day. First, they do not know the author personally. It is indeed important to become acquainted with the author of the Bible (God) in order to understand just how valuable the Bible can be. 1 Corinthians 1:18 tells us that unbelievers will find the Bible to be foolishness. They are blinded by the god of this world—Satan (2 Corinthians 4:4). When we have a close relationship with God, His words become our lifeline, and the Holy Spirit helps us to understand the words.

The second reason people have difficulty reading the Bible is that it is an uncomfortable experience for them. It tells the truth about the depravity of mankind and it gives the only solution for getting rid of this depravity—Jesus Christ. "The Bible is in one sense the most difficult of books to read, because no other book in the world exposes our true motives or judges our innermost thoughts like the Bible. Thus reading the Bible can be a very uncomfortable experience. That's why so many have tried to discredit it."[1] I've heard it said that many people criticize the Bible because it criticizes them.

The Bible makes us look at ourselves the way God looks at us without Jesus, and that gives us an uneasy feeling. The Bible serves as a yardstick that measures our lives, and a spiritual mirror that shows us as we really are, without mask and makeup. It shows us the truth, and people don't like to be confronted with the truth, so they find it hard to read the Bible.

The Bible has trustworthy knowledge that brings us face-to-face with God. It teaches us God's spiritual law and His enduring promise that sustains our Christian life. The Bible tells us about the love and grace of God. Ephesians 6:17 tells us that the Bible is a sword in man's fight against temptation. Jesus Christ gave us an example of how to overcome the devil's temptations by using the Word of God. When He was tempted in the wilderness, Jesus defeated Satan all three times by using the Word of God. Psalm 119:11 states, "Thy word have I hid in mine heart that I might not sin against thee." The Bible serves as a spiritual and moral looking glass (James 1:23-25) that lets us see our spiritual condition. It reveals the plan of redemption of the human race through Christ Jesus, and helps us to witness effectively for Christ. The Bible also serves as the spiritual food that nourishes and sustains our Christian life. It is truly our lifeline.

For ages, the Bible has been subjected to skeptics who deny it is really the Word of God, atheists who deny the existence of God altogether, others who have tried to change it or dismiss parts of it, those who have tried to distort the Word to challenge its authenticity, and still others who say the Bible is outdated and irrelevant to modern Christians.

Through it all, the Bible has survived, and the enduring promises remain unchanged even to this day. I am convinced, and I believe with all my heart, that thousands of years from now (if Jesus Christ hasn't returned for Christians by then), the Word of God will still be giving people hope for a better world, and will still be bringing them in contact with the genuine and real Person of Christ Jesus.

There are many religions in this world, each with its own sacred writing. Moslems have the Koran, Buddhists the Tripitaka (three baskets), Hindus have the holy Vedas, Upanishads, and Bhagavad Gita. We have the Word of God, the Holy Bible.

The Bible is very different from other sacred writings. It is the only book that tells about the depravity of man, the need for rebirth in Christ, and the promise of redemption through Christ Jesus. The Bible makes it clear that man can do nothing on his own about peace, hope for the future, and everlasting life. These come from Christ Jesus. The Bible also teaches us that the only chance this universe has for salvation is through Jesus Christ. Now, more than ever, we need to draw closer to Him. We can do this through a personal walk with Him, and through the Word.

Possessing the Word of God in the Bible, what are we to do with it? We must receive it, study it, and obey it.

Receive It

We must first believe in our hearts that it is truly the Word of God. 2 Timothy 3:16–17 tells us, "All scripture is given by inspiration of God, and is profitable for doctrine, for reproof, for correction, for instruction in righteousness: that the man of God may be perfect, thoroughly furnished unto all good works." We must have faith and trust in the Word of God, and receive it wholeheartedly (John 17:8).

We must receive it regularly from godly teachers and pastors, Bible study groups, and other cell groups. We can receive it through Christian music, books, tapes, television, radio, seminars, and conferences. Paul tells us in Romans 10:17, "So then faith cometh by hearing, and hearing by the Word of God." We must receive the Bible as the true Word of God.

"Do not say, 'I'd like to believe the Gospel, but I can't. My intellect won't let me.' The kind of belief here in view is belief with the will—the part of you that makes decisions. Your intellect grasps the facts of the Gospel, and your will believes them. Don't insist on understanding the Gospel before you believe it. Understanding may come later, but don't forget that God, being infinite, is beyond the comprehension of your human mind."[2] Accept the Gospel wholeheartedly, in spite of your lack of understanding.

Study It

After you've received the Bible, you must study it. Don't just skim through it or pick chapters at random to read. Studying the Bible involves a careful investigation of the Scriptures. Start with a book in the Bible and read one chapter at a time until you complete the Bible. Be consistent. Set aside a time to read the Bible daily. Make it a lifetime obligation. Take notes and use a concordance, if necessary. Psalm 119:11 admonishes us to hide the Scriptures in our hearts so that we do not sin. This implies memorizing key portions of the Bible and securing them in our hearts to use at a time when we feel tried or tested.

Proverbs 7:2–3 states: "Keep my commandments and live; and my law as the apple of thine eye. Bind them upon thy fingers, write them upon the table of thine heart." When we memorize the Scriptures, it helps us in our Christian growth, enables us to pray more effectively, gives us victory over sins and over Satan, and assists us in our witnessing to others.

As you read the Scriptures, ask the Holy Spirit to help you understand it better. Meditate on it and reflect on what you've read. What lesson is God trying to teach you? How can you use this passage to change lives? What message is being relayed? After reading the Scriptures, have a time of prayer and worship. (See chapter 34 for prayer and worship.)

Bible study provides a time of fellowship with God so that we can allow Him to speak to us. Sometimes, we are busy doing things *for* Him instead of *with* Him. Bible study provides a time for us to be better acquainted with the Person of Jesus Christ, and to allow the Holy Spirit to minister to us. It also provides for our spiritual replenishment and strength to survive whatever pressures we experience that day.

Wonderful and exciting things start to happen in our lives when we commit ourselves to regular time alone with God each day, reading the Word and praying. We grow and flourish, and the time spent in communion with God will be reflected throughout the day in whatever we do and wherever we are.

Obey It

It is not enough that we receive the Bible and study it, we must also obey it. 1 Samuel 15:22 tells us: " . . . hath the Lord as great delight in burnt offerings and sacrifices, as in obeying the voice of the Lord? Behold, to obey is better than sacrifices, and to hearken than the fat of rams." Friends, obedience to God and His Word is much more important than the "good things" we do. Too many people think that they can work out their own salvation through personal sacrifices, acts of generosity, by giving their money and possessions to the poor, by helping starving people in faraway countries, or by trying to "save the earth." All of these acts are wonderful, honorable, and commendable, but the prophet Isaiah warns us that our righteous acts are like filthy rags (Isaiah 64:6). All our actions (even the very best) are not acceptable in the eyes of God if we have sin in our lives. Our sins separate us from God and make us unfit to stand before Him.

Obedience to God involves genuine repentance and living a life of purity. These are hallmarks to genuine repentance. Obedience to God brings about changed attitudes toward Jesus Christ and toward sin, salvation, and daily issues in our lives like lying, the use of filthy language, our relationships with others, and our reactions to anger and other spiritual struggles. It is also evidenced by changed desires and a hatred of sin.

The second thing involved in obedience is living a life of purity. This is very difficult, especially in a sinful and immoral world. We need the work of the Holy Spirit and the Word of God daily in our lives to cleanse us and help us to live a pure life. Paul advises us to present our bodies "a living sacrifice, holy, acceptable unto God, which is your reasonable service" (Romans 12:1–2), and not to be conformed to this world, but to be transformed by the renewing of our minds so that we may prove the good and acceptable and perfect will of God.

Conforming to this world implies seeking to achieve the world's standard of living. We adopt its customs and values, which are almost always at odds with God's values. Psalm 106:35–39 describes what happens to us when we conform to this world's value system: We mingle with non-believers and become like them. However, in 2 Corinthians 6:17, we are counseled, "Wherefore, come out from among them, and be ye separate, saith the Lord, and touch not the unclean thing, and I will receive you."

This doesn't mean we should have nothing to do with non-believers. It means that when people look at us, they should see a difference between us and the world. We should talk differently, think, walk, and look different from people of the world. God has set us apart to bring praise and glory to Him through the life we live. Our obedience to God and His Word makes it easy to live the life He expects of us.

As Christian caregivers, we must live what we preach. This <u>is</u> obedience. Nothing is gained by someone saying he is a Christian, then not living what he preaches. Our patients, their families, and our coworkers <u>must</u> see in us what we preach. If you preach salvation through Christ Jesus, do you have a personal relationship with Him, yourself? If you preach love, do you love other people the way the Bible instructs us to do? If you preach forgiveness, have you truly forgiven those who have treated you unfairly? If you preach purity, do you live a life of purity?

If you don't do these things yourself, people will not listen to you. They will see right through your mask and phoniness. Actions do speak louder than words. Saying is passive, but <u>doing</u> is active. Maybe it's time to stop yelling that we're Christians and start living like Christians! There is no better witness to the power of God than a Christian nurse whose daily behavior bears out her profession of faith in Christ Jesus.

We must obey God's Word and live by it every day, not only on Sunday or on Wednesday nights, not only at church services or during Bible studies, but <u>everywhere</u> and at all times. We must be consistent and live a life of purity every day and everywhere. That's obedience! Psalm 106:3 promises, "Blessed are they that keep judgment and he that doeth righteousness at all times."

Thorough handwashing protects us and the patients we serve from infection by deadly germs. Living by the Word of God protects us from infection by the ways of the world, which are too often the opposite of the ways of the Lord.

Like the ritual cleansing in the Jewish tradition, clean hands symbolize purity, the holiness without which we are not fit for the presence of God. Psalm 24:3–4 tells us that only a person with clean hands and a pure heart may stand in His presence. When we wash our hands, it is symbolic of the daily washing away of our sins.

Today, if your hands are dirty and soiled with sin, you must trust Jesus Christ and His Word and allow Him to forgive you, wash you clean, and make you spotless and fit to stand before the Father. When He washes your sins away, you exchange your "filthy rags" for robes of righteousness, and you are then ready to appear in God's presence, unashamed. "Draw nigh to God and he will draw nigh to you. Cleanse your hands, ye sinners; and purify your hearts, ye double minded" (James 4:8).

Prayer: God, help me to delight in your Word. Help me to receive it, study it, and obey it every day. Let me practice what I preach. When people look at me, let them see the Living Christ. And each day as I read Your Word, reveal to me Your will for my life. Amen.

Thought: We read and learn the Word of God to fix it firmly in our heart; and when we act upon that Word, its truth from us will not depart.

—Dennis J. DeHaan

Notes

1. Robert Wells, *Prescription for Living,* (San Bernardino, CA: Here's Life Publishers, Inc., 1983), p. 59.
2. Francis Breisch, et al., *Facing Today's Problems* (Wheaton, IL: Scripture Press Publications, 1970), p. 23.

Proverbs 30:8—Remove far from me vanity and lies: give me neither poverty nor riches; feed me with food convenient for me.

7
Nutrition

More than any other generation in history, this generation is aware of the importance of physical fitness. Food is basic for life and the most important role of food is to nourish the physical body.

There is no question about the role a well-balanced diet plays in our well-being. "We learn from responsible sources that our nation's diet is the direct cause, or a significant contributing cause of numerous debilitating conditions."[1] Among these conditions are diabetes, hypoglycemia, high blood pressure and other coronary problems, weight problems, mental/emotional behavior problems, and even cancer. As nurses, we see many patients who are in the hospital or doctor's office because of the effect of dietary insufficiencies on their health.

We have learned from responsible sources that good nutrition, healthy habits, and a positive outlook on life help keep the body and mind in sound condition, but we are more than body and mind. We have a spirit which will live forever. Don't get me wrong, it is okay to want to take good care of the body and mind. But we must also be concerned with the care of the spirit. Just as our physical bodies are strengthened by what we eat and drink, our spiritual well-being depends upon what we feed our minds. As the saying goes, "We are what we eat." This is true, spiritually, too.

The spiritual menu is the Word of God. It is nourishment for the soul. The objective of our time of devotion or our personal time with the Lord should be to seek nourishment from the Word of God, to get better acquainted with the Person of Christ, and to know His divine plan for our lives. Jesus tells us, "I am that bread of life" (John 6:48).

Jesus Christ urges us to satisfy the deep hunger inside of us— the hunger that three full meals a day cannot fill. He wants us to be healthy, well-fed Christians who are enjoying the many blessings promised in the Bible, and he wants us to spread these blessings to others with whom we come in contact each day.

The Bible assures us that if we hunger and thirst for righteousness, we will receive it. God does not force the spiritual "food" on us. We must desire it above anything else. Just as the need for physical food causes us to crave something to eat, so our need for spiritual fulfillment and our need for the Lord lead us to crave the Word of God.

1 Peter 2:2 tells us, "As newborn babes, desire the sincere milk of the Word that ye may grow thereby." Milk is the food of newborn babies, and the "milk of the Word" is food for babes in Christ, or people who have just been born again. The milk of the Word makes them grow, but as they grow in Christ the milk is no longer sufficient. Just as an infant weans to solid food, there comes a time when growing Christians need to wean from the "milk of the Word" to "solid food."

Physically, no one is born fully grown. We are just children growing into adulthood. In the same way, we were not born again into full-grown Christians. We are first spiritual babies, then we grow into spiritual men and women.

Nothing is sadder than a child who cannot grow and who remains physically or mentally stunted; but, unlike the physically and mentally challenged, one who is spiritually underdeveloped is that way, voluntarily. It's a choice of "diet."

God loves and cares for us just the way we are, but His goal is not for us to remain babies all our life. He wants us to grow and grow until we reach our full potential as spiritual individuals in Christ. Who we are, right this minute, is only a fraction of what God expects us to be. He wants us to be *all* we can be!

We do not have to remain spiritual infants. Hebrews 5:13 and 14 states, "For every one that useth milk is unskillful in the word of righteousness: for he is a babe. But strong meat belongeth to them that are of full age, . . . " There comes a time for growing up and leaving behind the childish things you did as novice Christians.

Fit/Unfit

Physically, a person can be fit or unfit depending upon the individual's diet. Likewise, it is possible for Christians to be spiritually fit or unfit due to the type of spiritual nourishment we take in. There are Christians who are spiritually underweight and some who are spiritually overweight.

The Spiritually Underweight Christian

The spiritually underweight Christian is not taking in enough spiritual "food." He might be a member of a church which doesn't provide a well-balanced spiritual diet, or he might get some spiritual food but doesn't apply these lessons toward his spiritual growth. He doesn't have a daily time for devotions, and he spends more time in the world than in the Word.

Because his spiritual diet is inadequate, a spiritually underweight Christian's faith is often weak, shakeable and wavering. He cannot back up his testimony and is unable to take a stand for Christian values. He doesn't know how to witness to others about Jesus Christ. He often complains and whines about how things are, and is easily discouraged. Fear and doubt plague him and because his spiritual immune system is down, he is highly susceptible to "religious" fads that come along. If sickness or hard financial times come, or if disappointments emerge, our undernourished Christian stands helpless and hopeless. In cases like this, the devil has a field day!

Do you see yourself as being spiritually underweight? If so, don't be discouraged. There is a way out. You can be spiritually fit, but you must *desire* that change. Here are some suggestions:

1. Have a daily time of devotion. Spend time with the Lord. Get to know Him better and seek his plans for

your life. Read the Bible and allow the Holy Spirit to minister to you. Memorize portions of the Bible to use later when the devil comes calling.
2. Find a church that preaches the truth about Jesus Christ. Search well. Don't just pick one because it's big and beautiful and in a "good" neighborhood. Visit several and be sure to ask questions about their value systems and beliefs. Find a church that is in the business of winning souls for Christ Jesus; teaching and preaching valuable lessons that will convict, convert, and change people for the better. In short, find a church that will make you stretch and grow spiritually.
3. Find Christian "cell" groups like Bible study groups. These will feed and enrich you spiritually. If your church doesn't offer these types of support, visit groups from other churches. You will find these groups rewarding in your quest for spiritual growth.
4. Surround yourself with religious music, books and tapes to further your spiritual enrichment.

The Spiritually Overweight Christian

Here is a Christian who is actually being fed, but with the wrong kinds of food. What he is getting are "empty calories" of TV, radio, worldly books, magazines, tapes and movies. He might be getting a lot of knowledge about religion (all types of religion), but not much about Jesus Christ and His saving grace.

This Christian allows the cares of this world, the deceit of riches, and an appetite for the insignificant things of this world to enter and choke the Word of God and render it useless in his life. Worldly things occupy his mind and thoughts and drown the still, small voice of the Holy Spirit. He is preoccupied with his own pleasures and satisfaction rather than with those things that please the Lord.

The spiritually overweight Christian is too lazy to venture out and win others for Christ. He wastes his energy on worry and discouragement. He is usually sleeping when he should be serving, or he is too embarrassed to talk to people about Jesus Christ, fearing they will think him "too religious." This type of Christian risks heart problems and other debilitating disease.

In order for the spiritually overweight Christian to become spiritually fit, it is important to follow a rigid spiritual "diet":

1. Use dietary discretion. Watch what you "eat." As with your physical diet, you need to analyze your intake and your output.
2. Ask the Holy Spirit for discernment. Allow Him to show you what types of spiritual foods to "eat."
3. Change your "eating" habits. Acquire a new taste for spiritually nourishing food. This is a learning process. You must learn to change your bad habits and to seek out a more spiritual fare.
4. "Exercise" to keep the "weight" off. Spiritual exercise includes three actions:

   <u>Seek God:</u> You should not wait until you have time to be with God. You must make time to be with Him daily. Nurture the desire to seek Him. The best way to put it would be to "hunger and thirst" for His presence.
   <u>Listen to Him:</u> Listen with full attention. Block out other things that will distract you or make you take your eyes off Him. Fill your mind and thoughts with Jesus and the things that please Him. Receive the Word, feed upon it and allow it to seep in and soak your mind and thought.
   <u>Wait on Him:</u> Waiting involves anticipation and expectation. Expect great things to happen to you. Look forward to wonderful things taking place in your life as you become spiritually fit.

5. Maintain the "diet." As with a physical weight loss, you must stick with your spiritual diet or the "weight" will return.

6. Witness to others. Do not keep all that "Good News" about Jesus Christ to yourself. Tell others. It is not enough that you receive the Word. You must spread it around, helping others to grow.

The Spiritually Fit Christian

The spiritually fit Christian feeds his soul on the meat of the Word of God. He is healthy and well-fed. He has wonderful personal testimonies and can back his testimony with truth. He is steadfast and unwavering. His yes is yes and his no is no. He is disciplined, has energy, and is very reliable.

He is a true ambassador for Christ Jesus. He takes a stand for Christ and does not care if people think he is "too religious." He is able to defeat the darts of the devil by using the words he has hidden in his heart. He is growing and flowering spiritually, and his life reveals the fruits of the Spirit.

A spiritually fit Christian is really a joy to know. He enjoys the blessings from God and spreads those blessings to those around him. He is a powerful prayer warrior, and is able to teach, witness and win others to Christ.

We must all strive to become spiritually fit. We must never be satisfied with who we are in Jesus Christ. We must work to be better, seeking God's high standards and always growing to reach those standards. This is what God expects of us. He has the power to make us change for the better and grow, but we must invite Him to make that change. He never forces us. We must crave the spiritual food that will give us sustenance, strength, and growth and make us spiritually fit.

We cannot minister to others if we have neglected our own spiritual nourishment. We need to feed our spirit "soul foods" that will nourish and stimulate our spiritual life. God wants us to grow and reach our fullest potential as mature, productive Christians in His service. Receive the Word and feed on it. Bon Appetit!

Prayer: My Lord and Savior, I want to be a spiritually fit Christian. Feed me with food convenient for me. Let me be a blessing to everyone with whom I come in contact today. Let them see You in me. Let me be Your ambassador, to point people who are hurting or discouraged toward You. Thank You for Your Word that is my spiritual nourishment. With David, I say, "How sweet are thy words unto my taste. Yea, sweeter than honey to my mouth." Amen.

Thought: Some people wonder why they can't have faith for healing. They feed their body three hot meals a day, and their spirit one cold snack a week.

—F. F. Bosworth

Note

1. Ethel Remich, *Let's Try Real Food: A Practical Guide to Nutrition and Good Health* (Grand Rapids, MI: Zondervan Publishing House, 1976), pp. 204–205.

Part Three

Things We Face Daily

As she juggles her job, family life and other commitments, the nurse faces several important issues and struggles. This section deals with these issues and struggles, and offers support, encouragement, practical suggestions, and advice to deal with them.

> Psalm 107:19–20—Then they cry unto the Lord in their trouble, and he saveth them out of their distresses. He sent his word, and healed them, and delivered them from their destructions.

Romans 8:28—And we know that all things work together for good to them that love God, to them who are the called according to His purpose.

8
Stress

As nurses we have all experienced, at one time or another, significant stress in the workplace. In nursing, stress is a common occurrence, largely because we deal so much with issues of life and death. Stress is a highly individualized experience. Some nurses appear to be able to tolerate a great deal more stress than others. I must confess that I often tend to fall in the latter category. As long as we live in this world, we will be subjected to some amount of stress—this is a normal part of life. The important thing is how we perceive and meet these situations that cause the stress.

Stress is defined as strain or tension. It is a normal (sometimes even necessary) part of getting a job done, but excessive stress can damage a person.

Dr. Hans Selye discovered and documented the changes involved in stress. He defines stress as our body's response to any demand made upon it. According to him, there are two types of stress: eustress and distress. Eustress (the "good" stress) is the type of stress that a person actually seeks, looks forward to, or enjoys doing, like taking part in athletic events, exercises, the pain of labor and childbirth, and the tensions of competing for a job others are up for.

Distress, on the other hand, is the type a person wants to avoid. This type of stress causes a person to suffer, for example: separation and divorce, death of a loved one, losing a job, failing the State Board exams, or being expelled or suspended from work.

If prolonged stress is allowed to overwhelm a person, or when a person's endurance is so severely tested that it seems like she is losing control, this can lead to burnout, and "too much burnout, combined with too little application of coping techniques, can lead to clinical depression. . . . We do not want to eliminate all stresses from our lives, but we do need to learn how to better handle and manage the necessary stresses of life."[1]

There are several ways to manage stress which cannot be mentioned here completely, but there are practical ways in which to manage or reduce stress. Below are three of those ways that have worked for me in some of the most stressful experiences in my life. They are:

1. Be aware of the personal presence of God.
2. Do practical things that reduce stress.
3. Find a support system.

The Presence of God

Be aware of the personal presence of God, the Father. It is very good to know that He is always present, not only in my "mountain" experiences, but also in my valleys. You know, stress can be a valley in our lives. Hebrews 13:5b tells us that He promises to never leave us or forsake us. His presence is ever near us, leading, helping and caring for us. What a wonderful feeling it gives me to know that my Father, the Almighty and all-knowing God, is in control. The Bible doesn't say we won't have stresses in our lives, but that He won't desert us when we go through those stressful situations.

God understands stress. Let Him be your "stress absorber." Through your time of meditation, prayer and worship, draw closer to Him and trust Him to help you to go through that particular situation and come through with flying colors. 1 Peter 5:7 admonishes us to cast all our cares upon Him, because He cares for us. He cares that you are hurting. He cares that you feel frustrated and rejected. And He cares about what is taking place in your life right now. As 2 Chronicles 20:15 tells us, "For the battle is not yours, but God's." Don't be afraid. Give it to Him. Give it <u>all</u> to Him.

Reduce Stress

Reducing stress involves taking care of yourself physically, mentally and spiritually. One way to reduce stress is through maintaining a well-balanced diet and exercise. A balanced diet gives you strength and energy to meet life's stresses. Exercise not only helps you to look great and be healthy, but certain chemicals released in your body during exercise bring about a sense of well-being and in this way, help reduce stress.

Sleep is also important for reducing stress. There are studies that have been done that show the importance of sleep. Sleep is needed for us to function well at home, work and play, and it is also healthy for our bodies because it gives the body a chance to revitalize and replenish itself. In addition to sleep, rest and relaxation are also very important elements in the reduction of stress.

Another way to reduce stress is through a diversion—doing something that you actually enjoy doing, that will take your mind off your stresses, and at the same time give you a sense of well-being. These diversions could include gardening, needlework, exercising or visiting other people. "The diversions will be a renewing grace to you, a source of variety on the theme of your life, and a means of interrupting the unceasing pressures of stress."[2] Also, don't forget to play—we often forget to do that.

Laughter is my most favorite way of reducing stress. It helps me mentally to reduce stress. "Medical studies indicate that laughter releases chemicals called endorphins in the brain, promoting feelings of well-being."[3] Find something to laugh about, or find someone who will make you laugh and uplift your spirit.

Helping others is another way to reduce stress. We live in a self-centered generation and we are sometimes so "into" ourselves that we forget there are others who are worse off than we are. When we help others (especially others who are less fortunate than we are) this can help reduce stress in our own lives. We cannot be a blessing to others without being blessed ourselves.

Finally, we can reduce stress by getting closer to the Lord Jesus Christ, and by spending more time with Him. Allow Him to minister to you through His word. The closer we get to Jesus Christ, the easier it is to handle or manage stress in the appropriate way.

Find a Support System

You must find and maintain a support system that can help sustain you as you go through the stresses of life. Your support systems could consist of close friends, your family, workmates, or your church family.

The support system is necessary for several reasons. When a person is going through a stressful situation, it is sometimes difficult to think clearly, and friends can help you make wise decisions and choices that could help reduce the stress. Sometimes just talking with others helps make the "burden" lighter. It is amazing how much strength you can get from a friend who is willing to help you carry your "load." Sometimes all it takes is a good listener or a great affirmer.

There is no question about the importance of a support system, but there are some essential things to keep in mind. First, be careful about whom you include in your support system. You should include those who will give you sound advice and uplift you with affirmation and prayers. My pastor, Billy Epperhart, refers to this as "recruiting up" in your relationship. When you are going through stressful situations you don't need people who will discourage you or put you down. Also, be very careful that your support system doesn't become a "pity party" where you all sit and whine, grumble and gossip. These things will bring on even more stress.

"Isolation multiplies the weight of stress. Sharing with persons who care what happens to you and learning with them how to increase your resistance to stress multiply your capacity to bear the burden and carry the load. In this way, you fulfill the law of Christ that we love one another as He has loved us."[4]

I praise the Lord daily for my own support system. I am a member of a Bible study group at my church and I have never seen a more caring and supportive group of people. They simply amaze me. Whenever one of us is in trouble, whether it be physical, financial, emotional or spiritual, the "network" goes to work. One of the members starts calling the others, and before long the person in trouble is surrounded by loving, caring and supportive people, praying, affirming and uplifting her. Like white blood cells, they all rush to the "site" that is hurting.

It comforts me to know that there are people who care about what happens to me. I am sure this is the picture Paul had in mind when he stated, "Bear ye one another's burdens, and so fulfill the law of Christ" (Galatians 6:2). We all need support systems that will help us reduce stress in our lives.

Remember, stress is inevitable, whether it comes from family situations, job tensions, financial problems, or just making ends meet. If stress is allowed to overwhelm us, the end result is burnout and depression. The following chapters deal with these two results.

Prayer: Dear God, in the midst of this seemingly hopeless situation, help me to remember that Your promises are sure, and You will never leave me or forsake me. When it feels like the whole world is clamping down on me, remind me of Your love that brought You to earth to take my place. Let me cling to You and be able to say with Martin Luther:

A mighty fortress is our God
A bulwark never failing;

Thank You for your steadfast love and grace. Amen.

Thoughts: The church is not a gallery for the exhibit of eminent Christians but a school for the education of imperfect ones, a nursery for the care of weak ones, a hospital for the healing of those who need assiduous care.

—Henry W. Beecher

If you would lift me, you must be on higher ground.

—Emerson

Notes

1. Frank Minirth, M.D., et al., *The Stress Factor* (Chicago, IL: Northfield Publishing, 1992), p. 14.
2. Wayne Oates, *Managing Your Stress* (Philadelphia, PA: Fortress Press, 1985), pp. 56–57.
3. Minirth et al., *The Stress Factor,* p. 132.
4. Ibid., p. 510.

2 Thessalonians 3:13—But ye, brethren, be not weary in well doing.

9
Burnout

The term burnout was invented in the early 1960s by a psychoanalyst named Dr. Herbert J. Freudenberger. Most of what he wrote about burnout came from his personal experiences. He described burnout as "a state of fatigue or frustration brought about by devotion to a cause, way of life, or relationship that failed to produce the expected rewards."

Symptoms of burnout include hopelessness, emotional and physical exhaustion, boredom, frustration, rejection, pessimism, helplessness, paranoia, stress, irritability and depression. As nurses we all have some of these feelings some of the time. How do we deal with this? Some nurses cut themselves off from full participation at the job site, others clam up and withdraw from other nurses, and still others become very negative and indulge in anger, gossip and an unwillingness to listen to other opinions.

To find the cure for burnout we must first understand more about why it happens and what can be done to prevent this condition.

What type of people are more prone to burnout? "Job burnout is generally the end result of prolonged job-related or personal stress. The helping professions—nurses, doctors, pastors, social workers and therapists, for example—seem to be particularly prone to burnout. Why? Human service workers, who deal with their people's personal problems, are employed in highly stressful occupations."[1]

The last chapter dealt with stress and its effects on a person, and how this stress, if allowed to overwhelm, can lead to burnout. Because we know that nursing is one of those professions that is considered highly prone to burnout, let's look at what type of nurses are more prone to burnout.

"One of the tragic paradoxes of burnout is that people who tend to be the most dedicated, devoted, committed, responsible, highly motivated, educated, enthusiastic, promising and energetic suffer from burnout. Why? Partially because those people are idealistic and perfectionistic."[2]

A nurse who is highly prone to burnout is one who is totally committed to a cause and is eager to bring about changes, and because of her strong dedication to that cause, overextends herself, running the risk of physical and emotional exhaustion. She is hardworking and a perfectionist. She always seems to be in a hurry, sets very high standards for herself and expects others to meet those standards (an expectation that usually goes unfulfilled). The unfulfilled expectations lead to helplessness and hopelessness because she comes to the realization that she cannot force others to be like her.

According to Minirth, et al. (*The Stress Factor*), there are three areas of burnout: mental (emotional), physical and spiritual. Mentally, there is a feeling of hopelessness and helplessness, negativism, anger, cynicism, irritability, apathy, and depression, among other things.

Physically, "continued stress and burnout may bring on backache, neckache, headaches, migraines, insomnia, loss of appetite (or a never-satisfied appetite), ulcers, high blood pressure, constant colds, digestive problems, allergies, or, in the most severe forms, heart attacks and strokes."[3] Sometimes people who are burned out turn to drugs, alcohol and painkillers.

Spiritually, there is a feeling that God is powerless and that He doesn't care what happens anymore. This belief affects one's life as a Christian, because what we believe in greatly affects the way we behave.

Who are the victims of burnout? There are many people who are affected when a nurse is burned out: the nurse, her colleagues and coworkers, and the patients she has in her care. They all miss out on the joy and the potential of a person who can make great contributions to caregiving and health care.

Burnout also affects God because it prevents us from becoming what God wants us to be. It retards us as Christian nurses, and keeps us from carrying out our mission—the calling we have, to bring a living Christ to a dying world.

The good thing is that there is hope for a person in this situation. Below are practical ways to prevent and cure burnout.

1. <u>Expect let-down and plan for it.</u> Keep in mind that you are not perfect—no one is. Everyone makes mistakes (including you). Don't be so hard on yourself, and don't expect others to always meet your standards.
2. <u>Rest and relaxation are very important.</u> As my son Jeff is fond of saying, "chill out." Take time out to laugh and have fun with your family and friends. Take time off to spend on things you enjoy doing. Learn new things and do something good for yourself. This involves taking care of your body, doing exercises, eating well, and being able to sleep at least eight hours a day.
3. <u>Allow others to help you.</u> Learn to delegate tasks to other nurses on the job site. Remember, they too have a lot to contribute.
4. <u>Share your stress and frustrations with your support systems.</u> (See chapter 8.)
5. <u>Talk to the Lord about your problems.</u> He is the rock that will support you, and He will never let you down.
6. <u>Get involved in other activities</u> like Bible study groups and charity work. In other words, have other activities to fall back on, not only your job at the hospital, nursing home or doctor's office.

As Christian nurses we have all had stressful days when things seem to fall apart and it looks like God Himself has forsaken us. Don't give up—Jesus Christ knows what you are going through and His promises are sure regarding how to meet these times of crises. The Bible warns us to not be weary in well doing; one day we will receive our reward.

Prayer: Lord, I am tired and helpless. I have no one to turn to. Help me to rest in You and to wait on You as you

direct my path in everything I do. I remove myself from the throne now and put You there instead because You see the whole picture and can better see my future. Thank You for Your love that will not let me fall. Amen.

Thoughts: A crisis does not make a man; a crisis reveals what the man is made of.
—Warren W. Wiersbe

He who stands upon his own strength will never stand.
—Thomas Brooks

Notes

1. Frank Minirth, M.D., et al., *The Stress Factor* (Chicago, IL: Northfield Publishing, 1992), p. 16.
2. Ibid., p. 15.
3. Ibid., p. 17.

Joshua 1:9—Have not I commanded thee? Be strong and of good courage; be not afraid, neither be thou dismayed: For the Lord thy God is with thee whithersoever thou goest.

10
Depression

Webster's Dictionary defines depression as being pressed down, gloomy, dejected, sad; to have low spirit. It has also been described as a prolonged feeling of sadness, discouragement and an inability to get on top of things. Depression is sometimes called "the common cold of the mind." Mental health experts estimate that one in every ten people in America suffers from depression. The fact that we are Christians does not exempt us from depression. No one is immune to it. Some people will experience depression on a shallow level, while others dive to the depths of hopelessness.

Someone once said only people of worth and value have depressions. "Superficial people seldom have depressions. It requires a certain substance and depth of mind to be depressed. Courage is a part of depression. There is even such a thing as the gift of depression—a gift which enables us to be 'heavy,' to live with what is difficult."[1] Suicide can be an indication that a person is not able to withstand depression and has sought the fastest way out.

There are several contributing factors to depression. The first is a chemical or biological imbalance. An example of this is "post-partum depression." Other imbalances are related to levels of blood sugar and dietary insufficiency. Not eating properly cheats the body of the nutrition needed to function adequately. Sometimes, reaction to certain types of drugs (like sedatives or birth control pills) may cause depression. Psychological factors contributing to depression are unresolved guilt, unexpressed anger, fear of failure and a sense of isolation.

Symptoms of depression include collapse of self-esteem, insomnia, loss of appetite, lack of energy, doubt, complaining and worrying. Depression cripples a person and makes him withdraw into his own small world of self-pity and loneliness. When this happens, he might begin to think about suicide. He experiences feelings of hopelessness, despair, apathy, and sadness. There is a sense of emptiness inside. The depressed person usually believes he is unloved and unlovable. He truly believes even God doesn't care for him anymore. Depression is very serious and should not be taken lightly. The number of nurses and other health care providers who end their lives as a result of depression is growing.

Richard Berg describes depression as a "spiritual sadness." Depression affects the whole person. When we are depressed, all areas of our lives are affected, including our different roles; our relationships with others, including spouses and family; our work, play, and our involvement with church and community. We withdraw from God, as we do from people, because we believe that He has abandoned or rejected us. This withdrawal from God and others only serves to reinforce our depression. It is essential that we learn how to deal with depression. Below are practical ways to begin:

1. Seek medical help to rule out the possibility of a chemical or biological imbalance.
2. If your depression is caused by unresolved guilt, confess it and ask for forgiveness. Make restitution where appropriate and possible.
3. Express your anger appropriately. (See chapter 13 to learn more about anger.)
4. Get involved in the lives of other people. As it's been said, "Don't just sit there, _do_ something!" Keep in mind that idleness promotes depression.
5. Reach out to others for help. Make use of your support system. Look for people who will uplift you and encourage you.

6. Cling to Jesus Christ with every strength you have in your body and mind. He will never reject or abandon you. He cares too much for you to let you wallow in self-pity. The Book of Joshua (1:9) tells us that He will be with us wherever we go. What a wonderful feeling to have that assurance of His presence. Psalm 23 states, "Yea, though I walk through the valley of the shadow of death, I will fear no evil; for thou art with me; thy rod and thy staff they comfort me."

Even in the dark valley of depression, we can find a source of strength and courage in God that will sustain us in our darkest hour. Like the psalmist, we can say, "I will not fear" because God is near. Allow God to change your valley into an oasis overflowing with blessings that can touch the lives of those around you.

Prayer: Dear Lord, I am depressed. Today I feel like I just want to go to my room, shut the door, and hide. Help me to cling to You with every fiber of my being. Thank You for being there for me and with me. Thank You also for the courage and strength You give me, that sustains me even in times like these. Lift me up Lord, so that I can lift up others. Amen.

Thought: Life is like an onion; you peel off one layer at a time, and sometimes you weep.

—Carl Sandburg

Note

1. H. Norman Wright, *Now I Know Why I'm Depressed: and What I Can Do About It* (Eugene, OR: Harvest House Publishers, 1984), p. 140.

2 Timothy 1:7—For God hath not given us the spirit of fear, but of power, and of love, and of a sound mind.

11
Fear

Fear is a universal problem. From the day we are born to the day we die, we all experience different kinds of fears and insecurities. In fact, the first show of fear is the startle reflex in the infant in response to loud noise or loss of support. Natural fear is good and necessary for human survival because it nurtures self-preservation. For example, natural fear causes you to jump back when you see a rattlesnake. It causes you to be watchful and careful when you are alone in a dark and deserted area. It makes you take precautions and stay alert.

We live in a world that appears to be dominated by fear. People are afraid of the dark, of high places, of being bald, getting fat or being old, of spiders, mice, dogs, snakes, bad breath, strangers, and people of different color or nationality. There is fear of failure and rejection, and fear of the unknown.

Now more than ever, people are afraid of the future, and with good reason. Just look around you today; the daily news on TV and in newspapers is depressing. They paint a grim picture of what is taking place in the world around us. Husbands are killing wives, parents abusing children, nurseries being bombed, rapes increasing, drive-by shootings, drug dealings, terrorist attacks, civil wars, and new illnesses that seem to spring up daily—all of these things promote fear in people. Fear of the future is very evident in the growing number of people who go to psychics and fortune tellers to have their tarot cards or palms read. I know people who will not dare to venture out or start their day unless their horoscopes tell them what the day holds for them. We have become a nation of very fearful people!

No matter what our personal fears are, the truth of the matter is that unreasonable fear damages us physically, emotionally and spiritually. Heart failure, high blood pressure, stress and tension are all linked to fear. It makes us nervous and scared and causes us to perspire. Fear limits us physically from enjoying life. It immobilizes us. Our very lives are controlled by so much fear, we are unable to function as we should. In reality, fear keeps us in bondage.

Fear also causes emotional problems. It keeps a person miserable and unhappy. It impairs our sense of reasoning, making it very difficult to think clearly, and makes us believe people and things are out to get us. Fear isolates us from the rest of the world and makes us lonely and frustrated. It also keeps us from having the new and exciting experiences that make us grow.

Spiritually, fear causes us to lose our effectiveness as Christians. It makes us selfish. We care only about ourselves and our "safety." God doesn't even come into consideration. Fear also keeps us from serving God and others as we should. We cannot minister to others as God wants us to. It limits us and the gifts and talents with which God has blessed us. Most importantly, it causes us to not trust God or take Him at His word. We become scared and handicapped Christians, useless to ourselves, God and these people we have been called to serve. We lose out on so many blessings because we are afraid to step out and do those things that God has called us to do.

The dictionary gives us three different definitions of fear:

1. Fear is a feeling of anxiety and agitation caused by the presence or nearness of danger. An example of this is the feeling you get in the pit of your stomach when you see a man with a gun pointed at you.
2. Fear is a feeling of uneasiness: for example, when you have given a patient his medication and then realize that you probably gave the wrong medication or the wrong dosage, or the feeling you get when you are called in to see the Head Nurse.
3. Fear is also a feeling of a respectful awe or dread, as when you see a snake or a tarantula, or when drawing

blood from an AIDS patient and it splashes on you. Another name for this type of fear is reverential respect, the type of awe that we as Christians have toward God, which makes us want to please and honor Him.

According to 2 Timothy 1:7, fear does not originate from God. Since it doesn't originate from God then it must come from Satan himself. Satan knows the things we are afraid of, and he uses these things as tools to erode our relationship with God. He used fear in the Garden of Eden (Genesis, Chapter 3) and he still uses fear today, to ruin our relationship with God. And the way things look these days, he appears to be winning. God wants us to be bold, courageous and victorious Christians instead of scared, cowardly and fearful people, afraid to go out and about our calling. Fear is not part of God's plan for our lives. It is so sad to see a child of God who is supposed to be living a productive and victorious life, and is instead afraid to witness or tell people about Christ for fear of rejection or failure. What a pitiful condition for God's chosen people!

The good news is: *there is hope.* Below are some practical steps to managing fear.

1. Confess your sins. Sometimes our sins make us afraid to come into the presence of God. Just like Adam and Eve, our sins separate us from God.
2. Identify the specific fear. Realize that it isn't God's plan for us to be cowards, but victors. Understand that fear hinders our growth as Christians and renders us useless to His service.
3. Claim the truth of God's words. It gives us victory over our fears. Memorize specific Bible verses to use when you are afraid. Speaking aloud the Word gives you strength. The Word also controls the enemy and puts him in his place. Remember, the Word of God is mighty and powerful and sharper than a two-edged sword.
4. Take your fear to the foot of the cross and leave it there. Jesus Christ (who has power in heaven and on

earth) has promised to be with us even to the end of the world (Matthew 28:18–20) so we need not be afraid of anything or anyone. Only He can set us free from the bondage of fear. But this takes trust and faith in Him. We must have faith that He is capable of giving us that freedom and with that faith we can confidently say, "The Lord is my helper, and I will not fear what man shall do unto me" (Hebrews 13:6).
5. <u>Practice love.</u> 1 John 4:18 informs us that perfect love casteth out fear. Love gives us a new outlook on things, places and people.

    I once heard a story about a little girl traveling on a ship. The ship ran into a storm, and as the ship was being tossed about everyone became afraid and worried, and clung to parts of the ship for safety. Everyone that is—except the little girl, who was skipping along, playing. Someone stopped her and asked, "Aren't you afraid the ship will capsize?" "No," she answered reassuringly, "my daddy is the pilot of this ship." Oh, that we as Christians will remember that our heavenly Father is in control of our lives, that He knows what's best for us, and that only He knows the future and can better prepare us for it! The storm will come and our "ship" will be tossed about, but if we are anchored in Christ Jesus we will find a place of safety.

    What is your particular fear today? Is it a fear of people, or animals? Is it of high or open places? Are you afraid to tell others about Jesus because you are afraid people will laugh at you? Or are you afraid of what the future holds? No matter what your fear is, bring it to Jesus Christ today.

    Instead of taking pills, drinking, overeating, being sad and depressed, withdrawing from society or paying thousands of dollars to doctors, take a step in faith and give it to the Lord. He has great plans for your life (plans that don't include fear), and He promises peace in the midst of trouble and fear. We must trust in God and start enjoying real freedom and real peace in Jesus Christ. Then we can say along with the Psalmist:

> I will lift up my eyes unto the hills,
> from whence cometh my help.

My help cometh from the Lord
Which made heaven and earth
He will not suffer thy foot to be moved
He that keepeth thee will not slumber
Behold, he that keepeth Israel shall neither
Slumber nor sleep.
The Lord is thy Keeper, the Lord is thy shade
upon thy right hand.
The sun shall not smite thee by day
nor the moon by night.
The Lord shall preserve thee from all evil;
He shall preserve thy soul.
The Lord shall preserve thy going out
and thy coming in from this time forth,
and even for evermore.
—Psalm 121:1–8

<u>Prayer:</u> Lord, I am afraid of _____. I know I shouldn't be afraid because You haven't given me the spirit of fear, but one of power, love, and of a sound mind. Forgive me for not believing Your promises. Protect me today as I go about my job. May my life be a testimony of Your love and protection. Thank You for loving me even though I let You down sometimes. Help me to remember that You are in charge of my life, and that You know what is best for me. When I am afraid, let me run into Your arms for shelter and protection. Amen.

<u>Thought:</u> Faith and fear are opposites. The more of one, the less of the other.

—Alma Kern

Philippians 4:6—Be careful for nothing; but in everything by prayer and supplication with thanksgiving let your requests be made known unto God.

12
Worry

The dictionary defines anxiety as a state of being uneasy or apprehensive about what may happen. Worry, a mild form of anxiety, is characterized by mental distress or agitation resulting from concern, usually for something impending or anticipated. This chapter deals with worry and its effect on us.

Worry seems to creep up on us so easily. Just reading the daily newspaper or watching the news on TV gives us a lot to worry about. Inflation is a big topic that makes people worry. Will there be enough money to buy food and clothes for my family? Will the mortgage be paid on time, or will the checks bounce again? What about tuition, car payments, credit cards, bank loans, etc.?

Then there's the issue of crime. Will my family be protected while I am working the night shift? Will I be able to make it home safely, at 11:30 P.M. or 3:30 A.M., alone on the dark streets? Will I be caught in the crossfire of a drive-by shooting on my way to work?

In addition to inflation and crime, we worry about daily crises. My car broke down, how will I get to my doctor's appointment? Did I post my taxes on time? Am I getting too fat? Will people like me? Will I be late to work?

All these problems make us worry, and worry may cause physical, emotional and spiritual problems.

We know the effect worry has over the body. Doctors warn us that the health of our tissues and organs is greatly affected by our nervous condition. According to Dr. W. C. Alvarez, a specialist at the Mayo Clinic, "80 percent of the stomach disorders that come to us are not organic but functional. Wrong mental and spiritual attitudes throw functional disturbances into digestion. Most of our ills are caused by worry and fear, and it is my experience that faith is more important than food in the cure of stomach ulcers."

We torture ourselves when we worry. We lie awake at night picturing troubles we might have tomorrow. Someone once said, "Concern becomes worry when it is focused on the wrong day—tomorrow!"

Worry also causes emotional problems. It makes a person tense, jumpy and very nervous, and it spills over into people around us. Have you noticed that "worry warts" always seem to bring their worries with them everywhere they go? They aren't satisfied to keep their own spirits "down," but proceed to infect everyone else around with their "worry bacteria."

Worry attacks us spiritually. It is often a refusal to take God at His word. To put it plain and simple, we worry because we don't want to believe God. Worry causes the Word of God to lose its effectiveness in our lives. We are so busy worrying, we fail to acknowledge the fact that our Father God owns everything in this universe, that these things are at our disposal, and that we only have to ask Him for them.

When we worry, what we are doing is taking upon ourselves the responsibility that belongs to God. He sees tomorrow—let <u>Him</u> worry about tomorrow. As someone wisely put it, "God sees the end from the beginning." Who then is better prepared to worry about tomorrow, you or God? God, of course.

A child feels safe and secure clinging to his daddy's arms. All is well in his little world. He has no worries because his daddy is big and strong and can handle anything and everything. Wouldn't it be great if we could cling to our Father's arms and feel safe and secure? Too often we behave as though we don't know God is capable of guarding us, protecting us, or meeting our every need.

Problems are never solved by worrying. In fact the more we worry, the bigger our problems become. Matthew 6:27 tells us that being anxious or worrying does not add a single minute to our life span. And do you know that most of the things and issues we worry about eventually never take place?

It is not God's will that His people should be weighed down with the cares of this world. Below are some practical ways to keep worry away.

> 1. <u>Start to trust God.</u> Take Him at His word. We have abundant promises that God can meet our needs, and faith causes us to rise and take hold of these promises. When faith enters, worry runs out, and the stronger our faith, the more we rely on God. Faith gives us immunity against worry.

Matthew 6:8 tells us that God knows our needs even before we ask Him. He knows we need clothes and food for our families. He knows we have to pay mortgages, defray car payments and school fees. He knows we need protection. He knows about our jobs and about the impressions we want to make. He knows <u>all</u> our needs and He has given us abundant promises towards meeting these needs. Let us take Him at His word.

Matthew 6:26, 28 and 29 tell us that if God takes care of the needs of the birds and flowers, He can surely meet the needs of human beings whom He considers "more precious." 1 Peter 5:7 states, "Casting all your care upon him; for he careth for you." Our burdens and worries are not our responsibilities—they are God's.

Philippians 4:19 also assures us that God shall supply <u>all</u> our needs. It states <u>all</u> our needs, not some of our needs, or only the big needs. It states <u>all</u>. I like the use of the word "shall." It implies an act you can take to the bank. It doesn't say "maybe" God can supply our needs or "perhaps" God will supply our needs. He shall supply <u>all</u> our needs. It comforts me to know I have a Daddy who cares so much for me.

> 2. <u>Start praying.</u> Have you noticed that you tend to worry even more when you aren't praying like you should? I have. When I am close to God in my daily devotions, I don't find the time to worry. Praying reinforces our faith in God and His power to meet our needs.
>
> 3. <u>Start praising.</u> Let's praise God for the things we are

already blessed with. As the song goes, "Count your blessings, name them one by one, count your many blessings, see what God has done." When we praise Him, we are bringing to remembrance all these blessings He has given us and that He is willing to give us even more.

Praise also breaks the heaviness and anxiety that worrying brings. It uplifts and soothes the heavy heart.

    4. <u>Get busy serving others.</u> Make the world a little bit better for someone else and you won't have time to worry about your own problems. Service sharpens our sensitivity to the needs of others and most of the time, we come to find out that our own problems seem petty compared to other people's.

Are you weighed down by worries today? Bring them to Jesus Christ. Through prayer and supplication make your requests known to Him.

<u>Prayer:</u> My Heavenly Father, I am so worried. My burdens are beginning to overwhelm me and there is no one to turn to but You. I feel helpless and very scared. I don't know what the future holds, but You do. Help me to trust You and draw closer to You, because You love me very much. As that child, let me cling to Your strong and safe arms. Thanks for loving and caring for me. Amen.

<u>Thought:</u> Said the Robin to the Sparrow:
    "I should really like to know
   Why these anxious human beings
    Rush about and worry so?"
  Said the Sparrow to the Robin:
   "Friend, I think that it must be
  That they have no heavenly Father,
    Such as cares for you and me."
—Elizabeth Cheney

Ephesians 4:26–27—Be ye angry, and sin not; let not: the sun go down upon your wrath: Neither give place to the devil.

13
Anger

Perhaps anger is one of the most common things nurses deal with daily. Certainly it is one of those things I have personally wrestled with in my own life. Reading, researching and writing on this topic has been a learning experience for me.

Anger is defined as a state of emotional excitement brought about by intense displeasure as a result of a real or imagined threat, insult, put-down, frustration, or injustice to yourself or to others who are important to you. This activates the "fight-or-flight" mechanism in your body, which in turn releases adrenalin which increases the blood pressure, pulse, and respiration. This gives you a surge of energy which, if allowed to, can infuse your entire body.

People react to anger in many ways. Three of the ways are: by repressing it, camouflaging it, and by being hostile with violent bursts of temper. Let's look at each of these ways individually.

Repressing

A person who represses anger is actually convinced that he has no anger in his life. He will say, "No, I am not angry," when quite obviously he is. He represses his anger in such a way that he is completely numb to his feelings, but in reality has a great deal of anger buried underneath. This bottled-up anger becomes an unresolved anger which in turn "can lead to tremendous guilt, obesity, or insomnia. It can manifest itself in psychosomatic illnesses like backache, dermatological conditions, headache, gastrointestinal symptoms, and ulcers. Other possible manifestations are sexual problems and fatigue."[1]

In addition, there are emotional symptoms like neuroses, depression, psychoses, and a great potential for murder and suicide. We all have seen or heard about examples of this type of anger. Someone described as quiet, nice, and who "never gets angry" goes home one day, gets his gun, and comes into the workplace and shoots innocent people. That repressed anger finally surfaces in a tragic way.

Camouflaging

Camouflaging is the other way people react to anger, and there are several ways this is done. There is the "saver" who carefully saves up each little annoyance or grievance, until one day he blows up and that pent-up anger and rage comes out with terrible consequences.

Then there is the "don't make waves" individual who takes the blame for everything, even things he isn't responsible for, because he wants peace at any price. He never appears angry, but in reality is putting on a show, because underneath it all, he's very angry and can't express that anger.

Finally, there is the "silent approach" type who retreats into an icy silence. Where I come from, this is known as "keeping speech." He refuses to speak to the person he's angry with or to have anything to do with him. When asked if he's angry, he would deny anything is wrong but then grumbles and makes sarcastic remarks about that person to everyone else around him. This individual often has "psychosomatic complaints which serve as a means of dissipating the anger."[2]

Outbursts of Temper, Hostility and Violence

This type of reaction to anger is the type that pastors speak against in sermons. This type uses physical attack, hostility, verbal abuse, sarcasm, and harsh, biting words that cut the other person down. In short, he "blows his top." He might use emotional withdrawal as punishment and peer recruitment by turning others against the other person.

Now that we've looked at some of the "many faces" of anger, let's take a look at what the Bible says about anger. According to Ephesians 4:26 and 27, God allows us to be angry (strange but true). Even though God allows us to be angry, the Bible warns us to "sin not." If we allow our anger to cause us to sin, then this goes against God's Word.

God Himself expressed anger. "The Hebrew word for anger appears approximately 455 times in the Old Testament, and of these, 375 times it is referring to the anger of God."[3] Jesus also expressed anger. Two examples are when He drove out the moneychangers in the temple (Mark 11:15–17), and when He lashed out at the Pharisees, calling them hypocrites, serpents, and white-washed graves which appear beautiful outside but are full of dead bodies inside. Jesus was angry due to the misuse of the temple and the misguided values of the Pharisees, but He did not sin—He was without sin, the Bible tells us. He had the right to get angry. He was angry for the right reasons.

Anger is a natural, God-given emotion that needs to be expressed sometimes. Our inability to become angry (when we should be angry) can make us insensitive to the problems around us. Sometimes we go around with blinders on, unaware of or not caring about the injustices around us. We usually say, "As long as it doesn't affect me or my family, it's none of my business." Sometimes we need to be angry enough to want to bring about change, to take a stand for values we believe in. There is something very wrong when people fail to confront a wrong, and getting angry might be the beginning of taking action to correct that wrong. Edmund Burke puts it simply: "All that is necessary for evil to triumph is for good people to do nothing."

There is a difference between anger and hate. Anger reveals that we are alive and kicking, but hatred shows that we are sick and in need of spiritual healing. While a healthy anger drives us to want to bring about change, hatred wants to make things worse. Hatred refuses to reconcile. It distorts our thinking and destroys relationships, unity and fellowship—all the things necessary for harmony between people working together. Have you noticed how nurses who are bitter about something can never seem to keep their bitterness to themselves? They talk about it long and often, and as a result the bitterness spreads around the workplace like flu. When we allow our anger to grow into hatred and bitterness, we sin.

In Ephesians 4:26 and 27, Paul shows us how to deal with anger. He admonishes us to not let the sun go down on our anger. In other words, we must do something about our anger right away, when we still have the time and the opportunity. Nursing our anger and allowing it to turn into bitterness and hatred is allowing a loophole for the devil. The longer you nurse the bitterness, the more things you will find to be bitter about, and pretty soon the devil takes over.

Below are practical ways to handle anger:

1. Recognize your feelings of anger and evaluate just how angry you are. Be careful to not overreact to minor issues or under-react to major ones.
2. Suppress any action until you have thought through the situation. (This is not the same as repressing our anger.) This is the time when some people will suggest counting from 1 to 10. At this time, pray that God will help you see the issue clearly.
3. Identify the cause of your anger. What is it that is making you angry. Who are you really angry with? Be careful that your anger is not displaced. An example of this is—you get angry with someone at work, you go home and get angry with your child, and he goes out and kicks his dog.
4. Determine a course of action to take. There are several ways to do this. Confront the other person when necessary. Do it in private and if possible the same day. Don't allow your anger to fester into bitterness before confronting that person. Also be willing to listen to the other person's side of the story. Another course of action is to compromise when it is appropriate. You can

do so by saying, "I'll admit that some of it was my fault." The last course of action will be to just overlook the offense in order to avoid further conflict. In this case, let it rest. Do not bring the matter back to mind a week later and open a scar that is supposed to be healed by then.

No matter which course of action you take, it is very important to note that revengeful and vindictive anger is sin and we must deal with that sin as we would other sins—confess to God and ask for forgiveness. We should also practice forgiveness ourselves.

Paul admonishes us in Ephesians 4:32 to be kind to one another. Compassion and kindness drive away bitterness. The Bible tells us to express kindness to the offender (Romans 12:20). This is the hard part, but this is also what is required of us as Christians. Love is stronger than hate, forgiveness better than retaliation. Hatred and retaliation will be giving place to the devil. Let go of the anger and live!

Prayer: My Heavenly Father, I am so worried. My burdens are beginning to overwhelm me and there is no one to turn to but You. I feel helpless and very scared. I don't know what the future holds, but You do. Help me to trust You and draw closer to You, because You love me very much. As that child, let me cling to Your strong and safe arms. Thanks for loving and caring for me. Amen.

Thoughts: A Christian is more likely to sin by his reactions than his actions.
—Stanley Jones

Each person is responsible to God for what he has done with what others have done to him.
—O. S. Guinness

Notes

1. D. L. Carlson, M.D., *Overcoming Hurts and Anger: How to Identify and Cope with Negative Emotions* (Eugene, OR: Harvest House Publishers, 1981), p. 26.
2. Ibid., p. 22.
3. Ibid., p. 35.

Proverbs 16:5—Everyone that is proud in heart is an abomination to the Lord: though hand join in hand, he shall not be unpunished.

14
Pride

Pride can be negative or positive. An example of pride being positive is being proud to be an American or the pride you may feel being a nurse. Negative pride is arrogant self-esteem, and this is the type we will deal with in this chapter.

Pride means "to be puffed up" or "inflated." What a good picture of a proud person—someone full of hot air! Other synonyms for the word pride are to boast, to glory in oneself, to have a big head, and to be self-righteous.

Lucifer (or the devil) is considered the father of pride. The Bible tells us that Lucifer was not only good-looking, but that he had been placed above all the other angels. He was the anointed cherub and God's own light bearer. This means that he was an angel that God respected and trusted; but pride got in the way, and he became God's enemy.

Pride comes from the pit of hell and is the very root and essence of sin. In fact, it is sometimes referred to as the original sin. It is one of the quickest ways Satan uses to snare people, especially believers. Pride makes us to become impressed with our own abilities, and when that happens, we become inflated with our own importance and grab the glory that is due God.

A proud person is always boasting about himself, his possessions, and his accomplishments. He believes that he is self-sufficient and therefore never asks for help even though it is apparent he needs it. He has a demanding attitude and is concerned with winning at any cost, and it doesn't matter whom he has to step on to get to the top. He is always criticizing people and lacks concern for others.

Pride reveals itself in many ways. There is the pride of possessions. Some people pride themselves on the kind of houses they live in, the expensive jewels and clothes they wear, the exclusive country clubs they belong to, and all those things they possess. Somehow, they equate greatness with how rich people are.

There is the pride of intellect. In today's world, knowledge and education have increasingly gained momentum. It is no longer sufficient to be just a registered nurse; now you must be a Level III or clinical 4, or be a specialist in something, or a clinician in another. A B.S. in nursing is no longer enough; now you must have a Master of Science, or a doctorate. The pride of intellect causes many people to glorify themselves. Don't get me wrong, it's fine to want to further your education or become better equipped for your nursing career, but at the same time, you must be very careful that the glory for that education and advancement goes to the person who deserves it in the first place—Jesus Christ.

Then there's the pride of position; pride in what position we hold and how many titles we have following our names. Remember that God placed you in that position and gave you all those titles for a reason—to use them to His glory.

There is also the pride that some Christians have that makes them believe that they are "better Christians" than other people. Another name for this type is self-righteousness. They never make mistakes, their marriage is perfect, their children are perfect, their church is the only "true" church. They are just perfect, perfect, perfect. Know anyone like that?

The Bible tells us that righteousness is out of the question (Romans 3:10). <u>No one is righteous</u>. When confronted with the failures of others, be careful so that pride does not cause you to say things like, "I could never do something like that," or "I wonder if she's really saved." Paul warns us in 1 Corinthians 10:12, "Wherefore, let him that thinketh he standeth take heed lest he fall." We've all failed Christ Jesus in one way or another. Your sin might not be as "big" as the other person's, but sin is sin. Pride is considered an abomination to God, therefore, it is a sin.

Finally, there is rebellious pride that refuses to depend on God and to be subject to His laws. This type makes us believe that it isn't politically correct to obey all of God's laws, just some of them, some of the time. We no longer have faith in God or in the power of the Holy Spirit. As long as we feel sufficient in ourselves, we do not need God—then we become our own god.

This rebellious pride, and all the other types of pride, are an abomination to God. "Given enough rope, pride will eventually make us think we are capable of operating independently of God."[1] This is the devil's plan to keep us from depending on the power of God.

What can we do to puncture the pride in us, and release the air of arrogant self-importance? Below are some suggestions:

1. Recognize pride as a sin that destroys people and puts a wedge in our relationship with God, and ask God for forgiveness.
2. Put Christ on the throne in your life. Look seriously in the face of Jesus Christ—material things and possessions will lose their shine.
3. Give thanks and praises to God for all He has given you. Give God the glory because all you possess came from Him in the first place. James 1:17 states, "Every good gift and every perfect gift is from above, and cometh down from the Father of lights, with whom is no variableness, neither shadow of turning."

Possessions, wisdom, promotions, positions, yes, even beauty, come from God. Since these things come from God, what right do we have to take the credit? None.

We should be on our knees daily, thanking God for every thing He's given us. When we are thanking and praising God, we won't find the time to admire our "own" possessions, positions and accomplishments.

The Bible tells us, "By humility and the fear of the Lord are riches, and honor, and life" (Proverbs 22:4). When I think of humility, I think of our Lord, Jesus Christ, who came down from heaven to give His life for our sins; to take our place on the cross. He stooped to this lowly position because He loves us so much. Do not allow pride to damage the relationship He fought so hard to establish. Do not allow pride to dominate your life.

<u>Prayer:</u> Lord, forgive my pride and the arrogant ways in me. I know it is not Your plan for my life. Every day, help me to realize that I am nothing without You, and that everything I have comes from You. I thank You and praise You for Your unfailing love that brought You down to this cruel world to give Your precious life for me. Teach me to be humble. Amen.

<u>Thought:</u> Humility is an elusive virtue, because as soon as we think we've got it, we've lost it. If we don't know whether we are humble or not, that's a good sign.

—Angela Ashurin

Note

1. Ben Ferguson, *God, I've Got a Problem* (Ventura, CA: Vision House Publishers, 1974), p. 105.

Proverbs 14:30—A sound heart is the life of the flesh; but envy, the rottenness of the bones.

15
Envy

Envy and jealousy are not easy topics to admit to, especially for Christians. After all, we are not supposed to have a "jealous bone" in our bodies. They are two of those "silent" sins we are often guilty of, that other people might not know we commit, but that are just as detrimental to our lives as other kinds of sin.

The dictionary defines envy as a grudging desire for, or discontent at the sight of another's excellence or advantages. "Jealousy goes one step further, and wants to deny the other person that advantage."[1] Jealousy and envy usually go hand in hand.

Envy originated with Satan in Paradise. He envied God and this act led to his separation from God. Cain was jealous of Abel's sacrifice and this brought on a tragic end, a brother killing his brother. Jacob envied Esau, his twin brother, and used deceit to rob him of his birthright. King Saul was jealous of David's popularity among his own subjects, and tried to have him killed. Envy caused David himself to murder Uriah for his wife. Joseph's brothers were jealous of their father's love for him and sold their own "flesh and blood" as a slave. The list goes on and on.

Notice how many of these people were considered "men of God"? Yes, my friend, envy is a problem for Christians, too!

Envy usually grows out of our desire for power, position and wealth. We look at other people's wealth, position and power, and think, "I should have those things," or "Why her and not me?" Ambition, pride, greed, hatred and competition also contribute to envy and jealousy. These things cause us to take our eyes off the needs of others, and place our priorities on our own selfish needs.

When one of the nurses talks about how her son made the dean's list at school, and you think, "Why can't my son do that?"—that's envy.

When a coworker is nominated for the Florence Nightingale Award and instead of congratulating her, you say, "Who in their right mind could have nominated her?"—that's envy.

When your colleague is promoted to the Head Nurse position and you grumble, "I should have had that promotion, I am more qualified than she is!"—that's envy, too.

Envy is not merely wishful thinking. It is much more than that. It is being selfish and inconsiderate. Just like a child who thinks the earth itself revolves around him, we are acting childishly and immaturely when we envy others.

I will never forget the time I came down with the worst case of envy. My friend invited me to visit about five years ago. When I arrived at her home, I found that she had won the state lottery big time. She had won 22 million dollars! She was living in a big, beautiful house with a sauna, gym, huge swimming pool, and owned a brand-new Mercedes-Benz, in addition to other expensive cars, and with enough money to choke a horse. Boy, was I jealous!

The first thoughts that came to my mind were, *Lord, You know how hard I've worked for You, how could You allow her to win and not me? I've done everything You asked me to do, how could You give her that much money instead of me?*

At that very moment, nothing Christ had done for me mattered as much as the 22 million dollars! Isn't that a very scary thought? That is what envy does to a person!

Later, when I had time to think reasonably (and after a bit of convincing by the Holy Spirit), I realized just how stupid and ridiculous my jealousy and envy were. In the first place, I knew I could <u>never</u> win the lottery, because I do not play the lottery. Secondly, this person was one of my oldest and dearest friends. I should have been happy for her; instead, I sat there, feeling sorry for myself.

Envy affects the whole person—body, mind and spirit. It makes the heart beat fast and causes an individual to be "sick to the stomach." We become irritable and nervous, and lie awake at night, thinking and worrying about other people's wealth, power and position, and feeling very sorry for ourselves. Jealousy eats away at our insides like cancer, and if we allow it to, it festers into an open sore of resentment, evil thoughts and bitterness. Eventually it leads to depression, feelings of failure, guilt and shame. No wonder jealousy is called "the green-eyed monster"! Proverbs 14:30 tells us that "envy is the rottenness of the bones." How aptly put.

Envy clouds our perception of God and makes us doubt His power and strength in our lives. It makes us lose faith in His enduring promises. Envy keeps us in a rut and severely affects our prayer time. It hampers our growth as Christians, and ruins the relationship between us, the one who is the object of our envy, and God. It also clouds our perception of the wonderful gifts and blessings God has so graciously and generously given us.

When we envy others, we complete the act by saying negative things about the person, gossiping about him, or coming up with devious ways to make things difficult for him. In addition, we grumble and complain about how "unlucky" we are. All of these actions are unbecoming of people who call themselves born-again Christians. Envy and jealousy should not be part of our lives.

It is God's will to create relationships that bring about harmony, love, and unity. Satan wants the exact opposite. It is his very nature to stir up envy, jealousy and strife in relationships. When we allow envy and jealousy into our lives, we are playing right up his alley. After all, envy originated with him.

Below are suggestions on how to fight these sinful emotions that prohibit God's work through us and in us.

1. Confess your sins of envy and jealousy. As with any kind of sin, we must confess and ask God for forgiveness. James 3:14 warns us, "But if ye have bitter envying and strife in your hearts, glory not, and lie not against the truth." Until we can acknowledge the fact that we are envious or jealous of others, we will remain victims of those sinful acts. Let us be truthful to ourselves and to God.

2. Bring to remembrance the gifts, talents and generous blessings God has given you. Take time and list them one by one, then place this list in a place where you can see it daily. Take a look at the list every time you feel the urge to envy others.
3. Praise the Lord daily for His wonderful gifts, talents and blessings. When we are busy thanking and praising God, it is difficult to envy other people.

Today, each of us must search our hearts and confront our feelings of envy and jealousy. These emotions must be "aired" and gotten rid of if we are to truly minister to our patients and their families, and to our coworkers. Truth comes from Jesus Christ, and only He can set us free. Let us be reminded—we have to give an account of our lives before God one of these days. May He be able to say, "Well done, my good and faithful servant!" May we be able to stand before Him with our heads held high.

<u>Prayer:</u> **Lord, I envy _____. Please forgive me my sins of envy and jealousy. Thank You for the assurance that my sins are forgiven. Thank You for all You've done for me and given to me, especially my health, a great job, a loving and supportive family, my church family, my wonderful children (child), and my beautiful home. There is so much for me to be grateful for. Help me to remember these things the next time I start to envy others. Thank You for loving me and for calling me into Your service. Amen.**

<u>Thought:</u> Contentment: realizing that God has already provided everything we need for our present happiness.

—Bill Gothard

Note

1. Miriam Neff, *Women, and Their Emotions* (Chicago, IL: Moody Press, 1983), p. 61.

Romans 8:28—And we know that all things work together for good to them that love God, to them who are the called according to his purpose.

16
Disappointment

Disappointment is one of those things that each of us must face. Being a Christian in no way exempts us from disappointments. It is a part of life and we must learn to deal with it. The dictionary defines disappointment as the failure to come up to one's hopes or expectations. Ben Ferguson (*God, I've Got a Problem*) describes it best as "the sinking feeling we get when our plans blow up in our faces."

Disappointments come in two distinctive categories: in circumstances (when things don't work out the way we expected), and in people (when they let us down).

When the vacation you had planned for months has to be canceled, that's a disappointment. When you are refused a well-deserved promotion, that's also a disappointment. When you set your hopes high and in an instant they come crashing down, it really hurts, but the most painful disappointments come about when people let us down. When we put our trust in people and that trust is betrayed, it seems like nobody really understands how we feel. We can't help asking, "Why me? What did I do to deserve this?"

"Whatever the cause, disappointment brings the potential for hurt, discouragement, bitterness, anger, unbelief, and fear. The effects of extreme disappointment can linger with us for months or years, hindering our relationship with our Father God. That is why it is so important to learn to deal with disappointment constructively, and to see His purpose in allowing us to experience it."[1]

One major reason disappointment comes about is because we tend to put people on pedestals, especially so when they are Christians. We are tempted to say, "He calls himself a Christian, how could he do such a terrible thing? He should know better!" What we fail to understand is that no one is perfect—<u>no one</u>! The sinful nature of man often causes him to fail miserably.

The only Person who ever walked this earth and was considered "perfect" was Christ Jesus Himself. He is the only Person we should expect to be perfect and stay perfect. When we expect other human beings to be perfect, we are "looking for perfection in an imperfect specimen."[2] Let's face it, human beings are not perfect and never will be; that includes you and me. When we realize this, it makes it easier to accept disappointments in other people.

There is some good news about disappointments—they can be blessings in disguise. Disappointment makes us receptive to God. Someone put it simply, "Sometimes God puts us on our backs in order to make us look up!" How true this is. Sometimes it takes a huge disappointment to make us stop and listen to God. When we come to the realization that our own strength is not sufficient to get us through, it makes us dependent upon the power of God.

Disappointment also builds character if we allow God's plan to take its course. 1 Peter 5:10 tells us, "But the God of all grace, who hath called us unto his eternal glory by Christ Jesus, after that ye have suffered a while, make you perfect, stablish, strengthen, settle you." Friends, this is character!

The disappointments and hardships that come into our lives are not meant to destroy us or to bring us down. They are designed to help us build character. Our disappointments can be a source of great blessings if we respond to them in an appropriate way. Disappointments can become appointments.

As long as there are people, there will always be disappointments. Let's learn to accept that fact.

There are two very important things to note here. First, God is in control and He makes no mistakes. In everything that happens in our lives, God has a plan. You might not understand right this minute what those plans include, but you can rest assured that, unlike the Psychic Friends' Network, He really can foretell the future.

The second thing to note here is that because human beings are not perfect, "coming to terms with disappointment involves learning to deal with people's weaknesses. It requires us to develop patience, flexibility, and a deeper understanding of God's ways."[3]

Allow me to show you an example of how God changed a disappointment in my life into an appointment for His service.

For days there had been rumors around the Intensive Care Nursery where I worked, that some nurses were going to be laid off from work because of budget problems. I knew in the pit of my stomach that I would be on that list of nurses because of seniority, but still held on to that slim glimmer of hope that God would not allow this terrible thing to happen to me.

That sliver of hope disappeared when the Head Nurse called me to her office to give me the bad news. I felt like I was in a dream and that I would wake up and find it all gone. Surely God had forsaken me. He seemed distant and indifferent to my plight.

As I sat there in the Head Nurse's office with tears in my eyes, I began to take stock of my predicament. I had worked at Swedish Medical Center for about three years (the only place I had worked since coming to the United States). I had grown accustomed to the place and the people. Leaving this job would mean having to start all over again. I would have to first find another job, then try to get permission from the INS (Immigration Department) to work at that hospital, which would take at least three months. In addition to that, I was the only means of financial support for my family! My husband was a full time student, doing two master's degrees at the seminary, and I had an 11-year-old son. They all depended on me for food, board and tuition.

What could I do? Where could I turn? And incidentally, what lesson was God trying to teach me here?

As I sat worrying, Jane, one of the supervisors, told me that with my qualifications, she thought they might be able to use me in the Float Pool. Even though this was good news, I had mixed emotions.

Working in the Float Pool meant working with "adult" patients with "adult" diseases. In my nursing career I had only worked in the Intensive Care Nursery and Pediatrics. Working in the Float Pool meant sometimes having to work on a different floor every workday, and I hated that. It also meant having to leave my "comfort zone," for an experience I wasn't so sure I was ready or even qualified for. Needless to say, I was very scared. The future seemed very bleak. Why was God allowing this to happen to me? Didn't He care any more? Didn't he know I was scared?

Little did I know that God, my all-knowing Father, had special plans for me—plans I couldn't understand at that time.

Three days later, I joined the Float Pool. It wasn't easy at first, but by the grace of God, I learned, and learned, and learned some more. During the three years I worked on the Float Pool, I was able to work with patients who had a variety of illnesses; illnesses I would have never encountered if I had stayed in my "comfort zone." I worked with infants, children, teenagers, adults and the elderly. The valuable experience I received those three years of my career are too numerous to count. And because of those experiences, this book is possible.

I can now write with authority and knowledge from my experiences—something I couldn't have done if God (who sees in the future) hadn't removed me from my "comfort zone" and allowed me to venture into other areas of nursing. See how God meets our needs!

Are you going through a particular disappointment today? Are you thinking, *Where is God when it hurts so much, where is my Daddy?* It is so hard to "see" Him when we are hurt, discouraged, rejected, betrayed and in pain—but He's there, looking out for us. He gave us His promise.

You only see the here and now. You only see what you are going through this minute in your disappointment. God sees the whole picture—past, present and future. He is best equipped to look out for you. Whatever your disappointment is today, whether in circumstances or in people, allow God to turn it into an appointment for His service. He is really good at that!

In spite of disappointments you can be sure that "all things work together for good to them that love God, to them who are the called according to his purpose" (Romans 8:28). That group includes us as Christian nurses. We love God and we are called according to His purpose. Things will work out for the best eventually.

Prayer: Lord, thank You for disappointments. You never promised a world without pain or hardships, but it is reassuring for me to know that You are in control, even in my disappointments. Thank You for all the plans You have for my life, and give me patience to wait on You, because You know what is best for me. Amen.

Thought: I am always content with what happens; for I know that what God chooses is better than what I choose.

—Epictetus

Notes

1. Floyd McClung, Jr., *The Father Heart of God: God Loves You, Learn to Know His Compassionate Touch* (Eugene, OR: Harvest House Publishers, 1985), p. 83.
2. Ben Ferguson, *God, I've Got a Problem* (Ventura, CA: Vision House Publishers, 1974), p. 87.
3. McClung, *The Father Heart of God*, p. 84.

Romans 14:19—Let us therefore follow after the things which make for peace, and things wherewith one may edify another.

17
Strife

The dictionary defines friction as a rubbing of one object against another; conflict, as due to differing opinions. Friction usually causes sparks and the wearing away of one or both of the objects. So it is with human relationships. When two or more people come together on the job, there is often friction. Some of the friction may arise from very small differences. The result is strife. When we don't get along with someone in the workplace, it can be nerve-wracking, energy-consuming, and very upsetting. All the wrong juices flow, and blood pressure and respiration increase. It is certainly not a good feeling.

In the workplace, there are a variety of causes for strife. Stress, change, poor communication, dissatisfaction with working conditions, failure to get credit for work done, gossip, personality clashes, irritating personal characteristics, habits or mannerisms, all set the stage for strife in the workplace.

Stress

We are all familiar with stress and what it does to us. Sometimes, stresses from home can carry over into the workplace. For example, your child has a cold; the baby sitter calls in sick, and you don't have time to call another, so your husband has to stay with the child; then the plumbing clogs and there is water all over the floor. It's almost time for you to be at work, and the car won't start. By the time your husband fixes the car, you are already ten minutes late. You get to work still angry about things that have happened at home; you are not ready to absorb more stress at work. The thing is, your coworkers don't know you've had a bad morning and that you need to be treated with care, so someone says something and that anger and frustration from home spills out into the workplace. The stress from home, combined with the stresses in the workplace, make for strife among coworkers.

Change

Change sometimes causes strife. It brings about resistance. People are always saying, "Why don't they just leave things the way they are?" We can be set in our ways and change means we have to take risks and leave our comfort zones and venture out to new things. This in itself brings about stress, and emotions ride high. Yet, change is the lifeblood of the workplace and is necessary for its improvement.

Poor Communication

Communication is basic to human relationships, but poor communication often causes strife. Communication involves sending a message from one person to another. It also involves the message being received and understood by the other person. When the message is sent and received, it must be interpreted. There is usually strife in the workplace when there is a break in this procedure. At times, we don't send a message, or we might send a message that isn't received. On the other hand, we might send a message that is misinterpreted.

Communication can be verbal or nonverbal. In verbal communication, we use language to convey our message (or we write down the words). In nonverbal communication, we convey our message without using words; for instance, through facial expressions, tone of voice, signs and symbols. We send messages every day, but often our messages don't get across to our coworkers. Misjudging a statement made by our coworkers usually brings about strife. Sometimes, not taking the time to listen to others brings about strife.

Dissatisfaction with Work Conditions

When we are not satisfied with our work conditions, we sometimes express our dissatisfaction in ways that lead to strife. At times, there are not enough nurses to cover the shift and the workload is too much for one person. Sometimes, unfair work division by the person in charge, or the giving of a budget day (when the nurse is told to stay home because there are no patients to care for) can bring about strife. The feeling that someone has been unfair to us always leaves us uneasy. Work left undone for the coming shift or finding the work area untidy also creates strife.

Failure to Get Credit for Work Done

The feeling that all we do is work, work, work, and we get no "thank you" in return always brings about strife. Some people can see your faults more readily than the good work you are doing. We all feel the need to be appreciated, especially by our peers, but at times it seems like all we get is destructive criticism, and this causes friction in the workplace.

From the chapter on evaluation (chapter 23), we learn that criticism is good because it helps us grow, but a mixture of constructive criticism and praise does more for the relationship in the workplace than does criticism alone. We can learn to affirm our coworker. "In its simplest form, affirmation is identifying some characteristic, trait, or action in another person and giving praise for that quality, or action."[1] Affirmation encourages motivation and productivity. When I am praised for something, it makes me want to do even better. It makes me feel good about myself and, in that frame of mind, I want to strive to achieve more. Praise makes us more productive. Affirmations encourage us. "Encouragement is important to help each other feel good about ourselves. Unless our ego is healthy, we are incapable of helping anybody else. A wounded, poor ego makes us too preoccupied with ourselves. Our time will be preoccupied with trying to meet our own needs. A healthy ego frees us to care about others. When our own basic need for worth has been met, we can become genuinely concerned about the needs of others."[2] We ought to uplift each other with praises.

Gossip

Nothing is more harmful, degrading, or damaging to our relationships in the workplace than gossip. Proverbs 16:28 tells us that an evil man sows strife; and that gossip separates the best of friends. We all know what I'm talking about: whispers behind someone's back when they can't defend themselves, spreading confidential information, putting a person down when she is not there, etc. Gossip doesn't only destroy relationships, it goes against God's will for us. Gossip fosters suspicion and ruins characters and reputations. It also brings about friction in the workplace.

Personality

Sometimes, there is strife in the workplace due to a clash of personalities. From Hippocrates to modern-day philosophers, teachers, and theologians, people have been fascinated by human personalities and how they affect those around us. Personalities or temperaments can be divided into four groups: the popular sanguine, the powerful choleric, the perfect melancholic, and the peaceful phlegmatic. They each have strengths and weaknesses.

The sanguine has an appealing personality. She is talkative, cheerful, and bubbling over. She has a great sense of humor and makes friends easily. She has energy and enthusiasm and there is no dull moment around her; but on the other hand, she is undisciplined, would rather talk than work, gets angry quickly, is fickle and forgetful, and dominates conversations. She often interrupts and doesn't listen. Do you know someone like that?

The choleric is a born leader. She is strong-willed, decisive, not easily discouraged, independent and self-sufficient. She is goal-oriented, organizes well, delegates work, excels in emergencies, and seems to be able to run anything and everything. Her weaknesses include being too bossy and a "know-it-all." She is impatient, especially with those she thinks are too slow. She has little tolerance for mistakes and is unsympathetic. She is demanding and not complimentary, and may appear tactless and rude at times.

The melancholic is serious and purposeful, neat and tidy. She is content to stay in the background, but is persistent and thorough. She is a perfectionist and sets high standards for herself. She is self-sacrificing, faithful, and devoted. She has a need to finish anything she's started and loves charts, graphs and lists. But she is also hard to please, always remembers the bad things her coworkers did, and is not people-oriented. She is self-centered, withdrawn, depressed over imperfections, skeptical, and unforgiving. She expects others to reach the same high standards she sets for herself.

The phlegmatic person is easygoing and patient. She is quiet and peaceful and easy to get along with. She avoids conflict and keeps her emotions hidden. She is a good listener, and is sympathetic and kind. Her weaknesses are a lack of enthusiasm, excessive shyness, and a lack of self-motivation. She is fearful and worries too much. She is indecisive, hates change, hates being pushed, and sometimes appears boring and lazy.

If you look in your workplace today, you will find nurses who fit into these categories. Some seem to fit in two or more. Sometimes, these personalities clash. For example, if you put a sanguine with a melancholic, the sanguine, with her restless energy, would rather talk, while the melancholic wants to have the job completed at the appropriate time. When you put the choleric together with the phlegmatic, there might be strife because the choleric has little tolerance for someone who is slow or seems lazy. If you put a sanguine with a phlegmatic, the sanguine might appear to be too loud for her partner. All these different personalities, with their strengths and weaknesses, play a major part in how we get along with our coworkers.

Personal Characteristics and Flaws

It appears as if almost every workplace has its share of quarrelsome, argumentative, and meddling people who seem to carry trouble with them when they come to work. They appear to thrive on bringing disagreement and misunderstanding to the job site. Some are arrogant and proud and think they are God's gift to nursing. Others seem to be angry at the world. They don't smile or talk with their coworkers. They just do their work and go home. There is little or no interaction between them and their colleagues. Then, there are the busybodies who seem to know everything about everyone and go from one group to another spreading gossip. All these flaws bring about strife in the workplace.

Habits and Mannerisms

At times, our habits or mannerisms can annoy and irritate those with whom we work, which can cause strife in the workplace. Examples are: making frequent private phone calls, making ethnic or sexist slurs, wearing excessive perfume, telling off-color jokes, using filthy language, talking or laughing too loud, turning the thermostat up or down without checking the comfort of others, smoking, gossiping, selecting a radio station to play without consulting others, or personal untidiness. Because we sometimes have to work together in the same room, these habits and mannerisms can be sources for strife among coworkers.

There will always be disagreements in the workplace. Our goal is to keep strife at a minimum so that it doesn't affect the care we give our patients. Strife must not be allowed to interrupt the job we have been called to perform. The main objective is to see the job done. Personal considerations should come second. Below are some suggestions on how to reduce or limit strife in the workplace:

1. Learn good communication skills: Learn to listen to others and learn to convey your message in a simple and clear way. Avoid public displays of anger, resentment, and bitterness, especially in front of patients and their families.
2. Encourage and affirm each other: Uplift your coworkers by your words and actions. Give praise when and where it is due.
3. Learn to give and take criticism: (See chapter 23.)
4. Watch your tongue: Lies, gossip, and slander all put wedges in relationships in the workplace.
5. Be the peacemaker: As a Christian, you should be the person to bring about peace when there is strife. Don't start quarrels. Instead, learn how to build bridges between people and bring peace.
6. Learn to understand people: Try to understand how and why people behave the way they do. Read more about personalities and how people differ. Get acquainted with people of different races, cultures, and background. When confronted with habits and mannerisms, try one of the following:
   <u>Confront your coworker:</u> For example, tell her that you don't like or appreciate her ethnic or sexist slurs, or that her habits annoy you. Maybe she is not aware that you feel that way.
   <u>Learn to tolerate it:</u> Bend and compromise or move away when necessary.
7. Pray for your coworkers: Pray constantly and especially before going to work.
8. Be fair: Divide assignments fairly. Do your share of work and help others out when necessary.

When efforts to reduce or limit strife don't work, do not quit and go looking for another job. You might meet the same kind of strife there, too. Sometimes, you'll find worse conditions. Practice tolerance, understanding, and patience. Lastly, look closely at yourself and evaluate yourself. Maybe you are too thin-skinned and touchy?

Prayer: Heavenly Father, as I go about my nursing duties today, help me to not lose sight of my calling and my mission. Help me to be a peacemaker and an encourager to my coworkers. When they look at me, let them see a "Christ-like" nurse; one who truly emulates You. And when I fail (as I sometimes do), help me to acknowledge that failure and ask for forgiveness. Remind me of those patients in my care, and help me to not allow strife in the workplace to deter me from the service for which You placed me here. Amen.

Thought: I never yet have known the Spirit of God to work where the Lord's people were divided.

—D. L. Moody

Notes

1. Jim Conway, *Friendship: Skills for Having a Friend....* (Grand Rapids, MI: Zondervan Publishing House, 1989), p. 164.
2. Lars Wilhelmssohn, *Making Forever Friends* (Torrance, CA: Martin Press, 1982), p. 62.

2 Corinthians 12:9—And he said unto me, My grace is sufficient for thee: for my strength is made perfect in weakness. Most gladly therefore will I rather glory in my infirmities, that the power of Christ may rest upon me.

18
Fatigue

Fatigue is defined as a lack of energy, weariness, tiredness, and loss of a sense of well-being. As nurses, we have all complained about having no energy, lacking pep, or just being dead on our feet. After eight or twelve hours of running around doing chores and meeting the different needs of your patients and their families, your body sends you signals informing you of the need to rest. I remember coming home from work some days, removing my shoes and just throwing myself across my bed, not wanting to even take the time to remove my uniform. Fatigue and weariness are common problems nurses face daily.

According to Doctor Dwight L. Carlson (*Run and Not Be Weary*) fatigue has four functions: It can be a friend, a trial, a warning, or an enemy. As a friend, you are so tired at the end of a day's work, this helps you to sleep soundly. The lack of this kind of fatigue causes problems of insomnia. Fatigue can be a trial because it increases our susceptibility to sin. Chronic fatigue can be a danger signal: a warning to the body that something is wrong, or that some activity is too intense or has gone on too long. Lastly, fatigue can be an enemy. If Satan can keep us tired and weary, our work output is decreased, and there is restlessness, loss of joy, and a critical attitude. Spiritually, fatigue encourages doubt and depression.

There are many things that can cause fatigue in a person. Causes can be organic, physical, and spiritual.

Organic

Specific diseases can cause fatigue. Anemia, infections, and endocrine disorders like hypothyroidism and hypoglycemia can cause fatigue. It might mean a diagnosis of myasthenia gravis and chronic fatigue syndromes. Fatigue can also be caused by some birth control pills, nutritional inadequacies, obesity, and changes that take place in a person's life, such as menstrual periods, pregnancy, and menopause.

Physical

Fatigue can be physical due to overwork. Work that is done too long; for example, twelve hours of work, three or four days in a row, can take a toll on the body. Working two or three jobs at a time, or working extra for the time-and-a-half, can cause fatigue. Working too strenuously can also cause fatigue. Most nurses are the "breadwinners" in their families and they sometimes have to do a lot of jobs in order to put bread on the table, sometimes at the risk of abusing their bodies. The love of the "big bucks" can cause fatigue.

Other things that can cause fatigue are boredom, side effects of certain kinds of medications, insomnia, jet lag, and daily activities like drinking too much coffee, and doing different shifts within a short period of time. All of these things can overwork the body to the point of weariness.

Spiritual

Fatigue can be caused spiritually, by sin, guilt, and internal conflicts. Sometimes Christians wear masks to cover, conceal, or disguise their true identity. The mask becomes a shield to protect us from what people might think or say about us if they really knew what we were like. We want very much to be Christians and to obey God, but we also want to hang on to the things that go against God's will—to do this, we have to wear a mask.

Wearing a mask is like carrying a very heavy load around with you. It requires a lot of energy, worry, outright lying, and deceit. It hinders the growth of others and our own growth in relationship to Christ Jesus. "Masks are worn because we want to be known, but remain hidden. We know the futility of being phony. Yet the cost of being real is often too much for us. We think the mask of self-reliance, toughness, and rugged individualism will bring admiration from people."[1] We want to please people at the risk of disobeying God.

God wants us to be genuine and real. Pretense is living a lie. It also hurts our testimony, because eventually that mask has to come off and when that happens, it really is explosive.

Bitterness and resentment can also be spiritual causes for fatigue. They usually come about because of the result of some anger-producing situation which has not been handled properly. The burden of not being willing to forgive others can keep us in bondage and cause wear and tear on the body.

Unconfessed sins bring about anxiety and fear of being found out. That fear torments and tortures us, especially if we profess to be Christians with a calling. It is also unrealistic because God sees everything we do—so who are we hiding from? Unconfessed sins consume our energy and make us lack the pep we need to go about our calling.

Negative and critical attitudes can also be a spiritual cause for fatigue. As Christians, we sometimes like to act as "self-appointed" judges who sit in council against other people. We find fault in everything—our friends, coworkers, church, government, pastor, and our bosses. We remember people's faults instead of their attributes. Because we are unhappy, we try to make others unhappy too, and spend all our energy being pessimistic.

Trying to please people can also cause fatigue. People pleasers are individuals who feel the need to have approval and praise from others, no matter what the cost. We all have an inborn tendency and desire to be understood and accepted and therefore we strive to please others. This is normal. It becomes a problem when we make pleasing others our primary purpose in life, even if it means going against God's commands. People pleasers sometimes neglect family responsibilities, church attendance, and even God, just to please others. As Christians, our main purpose should be service for God. We waste valuable time and energy trying to please people.

The good news is that the prognosis for fatigue is very good. There are solutions that can help us regain the energy and pep needed to continue the work God has called us to do. Below are some solutions for fatigue:

1. See your doctor, to rule out organic problems and get treatments if there are problems.
2. Rest: Take time off from work to catch up on your sleep. Rest is defined as a refreshing inactivity after exertion; and relief from anything that causes a person to be weary, troubled, or disturbed. It is possible to rest without actually sleeping. Sleep is a state of unconsciousness when the body replenishes itself. Both rest and sleep are essential for physiological and psychological well-being. After a day's work, the body requires periods of rest or decreased activity in order to refresh and replenish itself. Without that rest and sleep, the body is unable to function properly. Money is important for family support, bills, and security, but your body needs to rest in order to function properly. Remember to avoid stimulants such as coffee and caffeinated soft drinks before bedtime.
3. Be honest with yourself, God and others. Remove the mask, confess your sins, and ask God for forgiveness. Honesty can be liberating. With the Psalmist, be able to say, "Search me, O God, and know my heart: try me, and know my thoughts: And see if there be any wicked way in me, and lead me in the way everlasting" (Psalm 139:23–24).
4. Practice forgiveness.
5. Stop complaining and criticizing, and start praising instead. When you are rejoicing, it's very difficult to be pessimistic.
6. Draw from the strength of God: As Christians, our

strengths lie in God. Isaiah 40:29 tells us, "He giveth power to the faint; and to them that have no might he increaseth strength." Psalm 27:14 encourages us to "Wait on the Lord; be of good courage, and he shall strengthen thine heart: wait, I say, on the Lord." We must wait patiently on Him to strengthen, uplift, and replenish our energy, and we must use our support systems and allow God to work through others to bring us closer to Him.

God's grace is sufficient for us (2 Corinthians 12:9). We don't need pep pills or prescriptions that give us energy. They don't satisfy our special needs, and they are temporary. If you are willing to come to God, He will remove or release that huge load or burden that you are carrying right now, and give you rest from the problems of the world. Come to Him now, leave your burden at the foot of the Cross, and rest in the loving arms of Jesus Christ!

Prayer: Heavenly Father, I thank You for Your strength that lifts me up and energizes me when I am down, tired, and overwhelmed. Thank You for Your Spirit that helps me in my weaknesses. Thank You for making it possible for me to say, with Paul, "For when I am weak, then I am strong." You are my tower of strength. Help me always to remember to turn to You when I need a lift because Your strength is sufficient for me. Amen.

Thought: When, sin-stricken, burdened, and weary from bondage, I longed to be free; there came to my heart the sweet message: "My grace is sufficient for thee."

—Author unknown

Note

1. Lars Wilhelmsson, *Making Forever Friends* (Torrance, CA: Martin Press, 1982), p. 34.

Matthew 12:37—For by thy words thou shalt be justified, and by thy words thou shalt be condemned.

19
The Tongue

How many times have you said something to someone and then wished that you could take it back? Very often, if you are like me. It is impossible to retract our words after they leave our lips; that's why it is so important that we are mindful of what we say, and how we say it. Our words are of tremendous importance. Words are truly powerful. Proverbs 18:21 shows us just how powerful our words can be—they can bring both life and death. "With our speech we can rob someone of his good reputation, steal away his trust in others, and undermine faith, hope and love. With our speech we can set brother against brother and sister against sister."[1] Our words can have a great impact on the lives of others.

The tongue is a spiritually vital organ; physically small in size but mighty and powerful. A Japanese proverb states, "A tongue three inches long can kill a man six feet tall." The tongue has the power to tear a person down, to degrade and belittle him, but the same tongue can also build up, strengthen and encourage others. What a complex organ!

God has blessed us with the power to speak—an advantage we have over the other animals and plants He created. How we choose to use this blessing has a huge impact not only on the lives of others, but on our own lives, and also on our relationship with God.

Someone once said, "The tongue, like the earthmover, can move a lot of dirt," but the tongue can also uplift a person's soul and bring happiness. The tongue can cause discouragement, lower self-esteem, bring fear, sorrow and despair, and eventually death; but the tongue can also give encouragement, help build a person's self-esteem, and bring comfort, hope and faith in God. The tongue, often described as evil and full of poison, can also be used for the good of man.

The Book of Proverbs describes the tongue as a sword (12:18), an arrow,(25:18), and as fire (16:27). Psalms describes the tongue as a spear (57:4), a sharp razor (52:2), and the poison of a serpent (140:3). Many other passages in the Bible describe the tongue as a weapon. This "weapon" is used to wound ourselves and others, and can be done in several ways: through gossip, lies, and filthy language, among others. Those topics will be dealt with in detail in the following chapters.

The Bible also describes the tongue as a tool that can bring health and joy. The Book of Proverbs tells us that words can cause life (15:4), can heal (12:18), can rebuild (11:9), and are like "apples of gold in pictures of silver" (25:11). Proverbs also states that words can cheer up (12:25), and can be like honeycomb, sweet to the soul and healing to the bones (16:24).

Words are so powerful, they can influence, persuade, and cause people to take action. Hitler's words incited millions of people to commit some of the most atrocious crimes this world has ever known. The Word of God is responsible for changing the lives of millions of born-again Christians who would otherwise be dying in their sins right now. There is no question that words can greatly influence our beliefs.

Go back and try to remember some of the things you said yesterday. Do you think God approved of your words? Did you lie or stretch the truth a bit? Did you give a word of encouragement to anyone or did you put anyone down by what you said? Did you use a "four-letter" word, or did you praise and glorify the Lord? Do you realize that God heard every word you said? If He replayed the tape from your life yesterday, would you be ashamed or approved by God?

Matthew 12:36–37 tells us that we will all give an account on judgment day for every idle word we speak. Our words will eventually testify against us or for us on that day. Will God be able to say, "Well done, good and faithful servant," or will we stand before Him with our heads bowed in shame? Our careless and vulgar words will surely come back to haunt us.

"God places a high value on words. He revealed His character to us through His word. Similarly, our words express the reality of who we are inside."[2] If Jesus Christ is alive in your heart, it will show in your speech.

If soap operas are constantly on your mind, it will show in your speech. If the only types of books, movies and tapes you are interested in are of the world, it will show in the way you talk. But if you spend time daily in devotion, reading and memorizing the Word of God, this too will show in your speech. "For out of the abundance of the heart the mouth speaketh" (Matthew 12:34b).

"Sticks and stones may break my bones, but words they cannot hurt me," goes a familiar verse. How untrue! Words can and do hurt us. Words are powerful, make no mistake about it. They can affect a person's life in a negative or positive way. Words of praise, love, encouragement, abuse, discouragement and negativism all make lasting impressions on the life of an individual. Words used in a negative way leave scars—emotional scars that might be ineradicable. We ought to be very careful what we allow to escape from our lips; someone's future might depend on it!

James, chapter 3, tells us that we can, and have been able to, tame every kind of animal in the world, but that we cannot tame the tongue. Even though it is obvious that we can't put the tongue under control, God can. David knew his need for God's help in taming the tongue, when he stated in Psalm 141:3, "Set a watch, O Lord, before my mouth; keep the door of my lips."

Only God can tame the tongue. God made our bodies, and the tongue is part of our body, so if something is wrong with it, we must go back to the Creator to fix it. Only God can tame the tongue and change it from a weapon that wounds, destroys and damages a person, to a tool that brings positive self-esteem, encouragement, comfort, hope and faith in Him.

Prayer: Our Heavenly Father, my tongue is a valuable gift, but I have used it in ways that are not pleasing to You. Forgive me for that and for all the other sins I have in my life. Cleanse my heart and make me aware daily

about the impact my words have on my testimony as a Christian nurse called to Your service, make my words life-giving instead of destructive. I say here with David: "May the words of my mouth and the meditations of my heart be acceptable in thy sight." Amen.

Thought: A slip of the foot you may soon recover,
But a slip of the tongue you may never get over.
—Benjamin Franklin, *Poor Richard's Almanac* (1747)

Notes

1. Mark Kinzer, *Taming the Tongue: Why Christians Should Care about What They Say* (Ann Arbor, MI: Servant Books, 1982), p. 30.
2. Chuck and Winnie Christensen, *Careful, Someone's Listening: Recognizing the Importance of Your Words* (Chicago, IL: Moody Press, 1990), p. 8.

Leviticus 19:16—Thou shalt not go up and down as a talebearer among thy people: neither shalt thou stand against the blood of thy neighbor: I am the Lord.

20
Gossip

It is so easy to gossip. Perhaps it's one of those sins that we all find the easiest to partake of and the hardest to break. The juicier and more spicy the news, the quicker we want to spread it around.

There are several things that make it so easy to gossip. We are naturally curious and we desire to be "in on the secret." It gives us a sense of importance that we know something others don't know. We find pleasure in the sensational and the unusual.

Gossip is common among Christians because we find it very easy to justify. For example, too often gossip is camouflaged as a "prayer request," and is sometimes tolerated as a weakness rather than a sin. Nevertheless, God takes gossiping very seriously. Sin is sin—only the consequences change. It is listed in Romans 1:28–31, as one of those sins we commit when we refuse to acknowledge and honor God. Gossiping seriously displeases God, and the Bible is very clear about it being a sin.

To gossip simply means insulting or putting someone down when he is not there to defend himself. Why do people gossip? Often because of jealousy. We think that by putting other people down, we are making ourselves look better. Will Durant wrote, "To speak ill of others is a dishonest way of praising ourselves." We use gossip as a sort of self-promotion. We usually gossip when there is unresolved anger and unforgiveness in our lives, and we want to spite the other person. Sometimes we gossip because we are afraid to confront someone, so we take an easier and more cowardly way out. At times we gossip because we enjoy hearing about other people's faults and shortcomings. We also gossip because we have nothing better to do. When work is less, people tend to find someone to gossip about. Gossip is easy conversation.

Gossip can also be used as a coverup for hidden motives. Many Christians are usually guilty of this. It usually starts with, "Let's pray for so and so, she is _____," or "I am concerned about so and so, his wife is_____." We say we care for and are concerned for the person's problems and that our motives are to help, but in reality, we are only sharing their problems with others.

Lastly, gossip gives us the chance to dump our garbage on others, usually garbage about our spouse, children, in-laws, neighbors, and friends. Gossip can be used as a defense mechanism. When you draw attention to someone else's problems they can't see yours.

Slander is a form of gossip. Slander occurs when an individual talks disparagingly about someone (even though he is telling the truth) for the purpose of dishonoring or disgracing him. The Bible also speaks against slander (James 4:11–12).

The worst kind of gossiper is the busybody. The busybody is probably the "first branch" on the grapevine! She is usually the one who carries the "news" along to other floors in the workplace. Other synonyms for a busybody are: mischief-maker, troublesome meddler, and one who tries to manage other people's business.

The busybody uses every available opportunity to probe into the affairs of others, and because she does, she always knows what is going on in other people's lives. She knows about others' financial problems, family quarrels, love lives and secrets. She has the latest scoop on who's doing what with whom, or to whom, or who said what about whom. The Bible also speaks against busybodies (2 Thessalonians 3:11 and 1 Timothy 5:13).

Gossip is not a solitary sin—it takes at least two people to gossip, one to speak and at least one to listen. The Bible doesn't only forbid us to gossip but it also tells us to refuse to listen to gossip. "Most of us probably think of listening as a mere passive event for which we bear no responsibility. The person who speaks must take responsibility for what he says; our part is simply to listen and decide what we think. However, this is not the perspective found in Scripture."[1] We are to avoid the company of those who regularly gossip, or at least refuse to discuss issues that might lead to gossip.

Even though gossip is one of those sins that are considered easy to commit and hard to eradicate, there is a way out. Below are some suggestions:

1. Learn to recognize gossip for what it is—sin. Confess it and ask for forgiveness.
2. Propose in your heart daily to not gossip or even stand and listen to gossip. Move away or simply say, "I don't think I want to hear that." A wise man once said, "You are lord of your tongue, but I am master of my ears." You don't have to stand there and listen to garbage just because you don't want to hurt the other person's feelings. What God feels about you is more important than what the world thinks about you.

    Sometimes it is difficult to avoid hearing gossip because we work together, at times in the same room. In cases like this, don't take heed of the gossip and most importantly, don't pass it on. Nip it in the bud.
3. Avoid situations that encourage gossip. People tend to gossip more when there is less to do. Remember—an idle mind is the devil's workshop. Get busy serving; that should keep you from gossiping.
4. Encourage other nurses. When we are encouraging others, it is difficult to gossip about them.
5. Be a peacemaker. Remember that you are an ambassador for Christ Jesus in your workplace. Throw water on the flame of gossip instead of oil.
6. Talk about Jesus Christ. If you need to talk about someone, talk about Jesus—it always works!
7. Take confidentiality seriously. Realize what damage you do when you spread information given to you by someone who trusts you.

Lars Wilhelmsson (*Making Forever Friends*) suggests that the next time you feel like gossiping, ask yourself these questions: Is it truthful? Is it needful? Is it helpful? If even one of these answers is "no," don't repeat the gossip.

Gossip destroys reputations, steals away a person's trust, and brings pain and humiliation to people. Everything you say about an individual should increase the esteem your listeners have for that individual. Remember, as Christians we should use our tongues as tools to build up, strengthen and encourage others.

Prayer: Lord, please forgive me for the damage I have done through gossip and slander. I know these are things that displease You. Thanks for the assurance that I am forgiven. Help me to remember the impact my words have on the lives of others. I pray that my conversation today will be pleasing in Your sight. Amen.

Thought: The only difference between a buzzard and a gossiper is that the buzzard waits until the subject of his attack is dead before he tears it apart.

—Author Unknown

Note

1. Mark Kinzer, *Taming the Tongue: Why Christians Should Care about What They Say* (Ann Arbor, MI: Servant Books, 1982), p. 51.

Colossians 3:9–10—Lie not one to another, seeing that ye have put off the old man with his deeds; and have put on the new man, which is renewed in knowledge after the image of him that created him.

21
Lies

It is very easy to tell a lie, but very difficult to tell just one. You have to keep covering the last one with another one, and so on, and so on. A lie is a statement of what is known to be false, with intent to deceive.

Lying is not exclusive to nonbelievers. Unfortunately, Christians often lie. Acts 5:1-11 tells us about two believers who were deceitful and dishonest. They were Ananias and Sapphira, his wife. They sold some land and gave some of the money to the church to help other believers, but then lied about the total amount that they had received for the property. They had kept part of the money but wanted the church to believe that they had turned over all the money. That was a lie.

Peter, one of the greatest men mentioned in the Bible, also lied. Mark 14:66–72 tells us that he lied three times about knowing Jesus Christ or even being with Him. We have all lied at one time or another, but the Word of God is clear about lying—we ought not to lie to each other. Lying goes against the very character of God. In fact, Proverbs 6:16–17 tells us that lying is one of six things the Lord expressly hates.

When Ananias and Sapphira lied, they were struck dead on the spot. God doesn't strike people dead anymore for lying, and our noses don't grow longer either, but some unpleasant things happen when we lie.

Lies ruin people's lives and cloud their reputation. Lies also ruin friendships and destroy confidence by sowing suspicion in relationships. Spiritually, a lie eats away at our testimonies, and dishonors God Himself. Lying is inconsistent with a Christian's lifestyle.

Lying is Satan's language. In fact, he is known as the father of lies. He has been lying since the beginning of time. When we lie, we are acting like Satan's offspring instead of children of the living God. The Bible tells us that God dwells with those who are honest and truthful. He abhors those who don't tell the truth.

When we were baptized it symbolized death with Christ to sin and resurrection with Him to a "new" lifestyle. Lying is part of the "old" lifestyle. The "old" self and the "new" self are incompatible.

There are several reasons why people lie. Some people lie to make an impression. They want to look good in the eyes of the public. Lying makes them more acceptable. Others lie so that they can appear spiritual. They wear a mask in order to keep a certain kind of image and they usually have to continue lying in order to uphold that image. Another common reason for lying is in order to receive benefits they couldn't claim otherwise.

People lie in many different ways. We lie by what we say, but we can also lie by what we <u>don't</u> say. "White lies" and half truths are when we mix the truth with some amount of lies. Exaggerations are truths that have been stretched. Even flatteries are a form of lies. It is also possible to "live a lie."

No matter what form or type it is, lying is not part of God's plan for our lives. When we lie we hurt ourselves, others, and most importantly, we hurt God. His plans for us don't include lying. We are to tell the truth not just some of the time, but all of the time. We must also be dependable and consistent no matter what the cost. Honesty is still the best policy.

Confess your sins and ask God for forgiveness. Without genuine repentance, we cannot live the way Christ wants us to. Repentance will restore a broken relationship that has been fractured by the sin of lying. We no longer need to play in Satan's backyard. We no longer need to be a slave to the sin of lying. James writes that if we submit our lives to God and resist the devil, he will flee from us (James 4:7). In the Name of Jesus, resist the devil and his lies and he will flee from you.

Prayer: Lord, forgive me for lying. I take You at Your Word that when You forgive, You forgive completely. Thank You for that assurance. Help me to read Your Word, and to pray daily, and fix my thoughts on what is true and good and right in Your sight. Amen.

Thought: The wonderful thing about telling the truth is that you don't have to remember what you said.

—Author Unknown

Colossians 4:6—Let your speech be alway with grace, seasoned with salt, that ye may know how ye ought to answer every man.

22
Filthy Language

A patient once told me that the one thing she hated while she was in the hospital was the food. She had been placed on a salt-free diet because of her condition. "Salt is such a little thing—such a common thing—that we take for granted. But how big it becomes when it isn't there!"[1] Colossians 4:6 tells us to season our speech with salt. Let's look at some qualities of salt.

Salt seasons food. Without salt, the very best foods would be tasteless. Food would be robbed of the pleasure it gives people. Like salt, our words should bring taste into the lives of people around us. Our patients, their families and friends, and our colleagues should be blessed by the words that proceed from our lips. As Christians, we season the world.

Salt heals. In parts of Africa, when a person is wounded, salt is placed into the wound until they can get to the nearest hospital. It is believed that salt starts the healing process. Christians are supposed to use their tongues as tools that heal and uplift others by encouragement, affirmation and clean speech. Our tongues should build up instead of break down.

Salt preserves. Before there was refrigeration, salt was used to keep meat and fish from decaying. Today, the world needs strong and dedicated Christians not only to preserve this world, but also to preserve the family, and Christian values. "Jesus sees today's world as a rotting mass of sin, and He has put Christians into this world to help hold back the decay. We are the salt of the earth."[2]

Another quality of salt is that it de-ices. "The layer of ice on the porch steps on a January morning is much like the ice-bound heart, hard as a rock from the impact of bitter experiences. Both melt beneath the application of salt: one, the literal commodity, the other, the salt of kindness and peace."[3]

Salt soothes. When I was a child and had a burn, my mother would put salt on it to soothe the pain. Likewise, Christians are supposed to serve as a soother or pacifier to people who have been burned by life's hurts. Our words should give hope to those in pain, to those who are bitter and angry, and to those who think there is nowhere else to turn. Our words should point them to Jesus.

There is no question about the value of salt and the importance of "seasoned" speech, but sometimes salt loses its savor (saltiness) and then becomes useless. One of the ways our words can be rendered useless is when we use filthy language.

Synonyms for filthy language are: foul words, profanity, "cuss" words, obscene language, and four-letter words. No matter what you call them, the Bible forbids us as Christians to let them even cross our lips. Ephesians 5:4 states, "Neither filthiness, nor foolish talking, nor jesting, which are not convenient: but rather giving of thanks."

Why do people use filthy words? There are several reasons. First, it seems like everyone else is doing it. Somehow it has become an accepted attitude, especially in the workplace. Filthy language has become so commonplace, it is no longer shocking. It's surprising just how tolerant we've become about this kind of vulgarity that would have at least guaranteed a mouth washed with soap a few years ago. Secondly, some believe that in order to show others how hip or suave they are, they have to use such words. Thirdly, some believe that filthy language shows people that they really mean business. They believe that it takes strong language to get their point across. Lastly, sometimes it's the only way some people know how to express their feelings.

Another way our words can lose their savor is through dirty or "off-color" jokes. Have you noticed that some of the best joke tellers you work with usually tell filthy jokes? It seems like the more filthy the joke, the more popular the person.

The saddest thing is that we usually stand there and listen to the filth. Why do we do this? There are two major reasons.

First, we do not want to appear pious or too religious. Secondly, we don't want to hurt the feelings of the individual telling the joke, so we would rather impress people than obey the Word of God.

Our words are shaped by many things: our past, our environment and culture, our beliefs, our relationship with Jesus Christ, and how mature we are in Christ. The world around us has a huge influence on the way we talk, but when we come face to face with the Lord Jesus, our speech becomes "seasoned."

Matthew 12:34b states, "for out of the abundance of the heart the mouth speaketh." Our words reveal what's in our hearts. One of my favorite children's songs goes like this: "Input, output, what goes in is what comes out." That is very true! Whatsoever we put into our heart comes out of the mouth. If we watch a lot of TV instead of reading the Word of God, it will show in the way we talk. We will start to talk like the people in the movies. If we spend most of our time in the company of people who use filthy words, we will start to talk like them. If we put trash in, trash will surely come out when we speak.

It is very easy to know a born-again, Spirit-filled Christian nurse the moment she opens her mouth! Our words do reveal if we are real Christians or if we are, as Dr. Robert G. Wells aptly puts it, "churchians." Our words are important. They reveal to whom we belong—God, or the devil. There is no "sitting on the fence" here. We either speak like the world, or the Word.

As a child, I lived in a dormitory. As a rule, we would have our mouths washed out with soap when we said "dirty words." I had my mouth washed out so many times I thought foam would come out of my ears. But I continued to use those vulgar words! It wasn't enough for my mouth to be washed—I needed my heart "washed."

A "seasoned" speech starts with the heart, and only God can clean a person's heart and make it whole again. It is so easy to say dirty words when the Word of God is not part of your vocabulary. Read the Word of God daily and pray constantly. Glorify God through praise and worship. Get busy talking about Jesus and His saving grace—you will find that filthy words will have no place in your mouth.

Also be careful of the company you keep. When someone starts to tell filthy jokes, or to talk "dirty," leave or let them know how strongly you feel about this. People will usually respect your wishes if they know that you really mean business and if you are truly living the life of a Christian.

Remember to season your speech with salt, so that your words can heal, season, preserve, de-ice and soothe those around you today who are in dire need of encouragement and a lift.

Prayer: My Heavenly Father, season my speech with kindness, love, and hope. Let me be Your ambassador to my patients and their families and friends, and to those I work with. Remind me daily of the impact my words have on others. Send me someone today—someone who is hurting and in need of a lift. May my words give him encouragement and hope for a better life. Amen.

Thought:
>   You are writing a gospel
>   A chapter each day,
>   By deeds that you do,
>   By words that you say,
>   Men read what you write,
>   Whether faithless or true.
>   Say, what is the gospel according to you?

—Author Unknown

Notes

1. Warren W. Wiersbe, *Turning Mountains into Molehills: And Other Devotionals* (Grand Rapids, MI: Baker Book House, 1994), p. 26.
2. Ibid., p. 27.
3. Jeanette Lockerbie, *Salt in My Kitchen,* p.5.

Proverbs 15:31–32—The ear that heareth the reproof of life abideth among the wise. He that refuseth instruction despiseth his own soul: but he that heareth reproof getteth understanding.

23
Evaluation

Remember the last time you went in for your yearly evaluation? After looking over your peer evaluation, how did you feel? Angry, hurt, belittled, rejected, ashamed or resentful? Did the back of your neck get warm? Did your heart beat fast, and did your muscles tense? Did you try to interrupt the head nurse or nurse manager in order to defend yourself, or try to explain why you disagreed with the evaluation? Or did you propose in your heart to get back at, or get even with the evaluator?

After you left the office, did you cry, grumble, tell others how angry you were, or how betrayed you felt? Or did you make sarcastic remarks in the presence of the person who had evaluated you? If the answer to any of these questions is "yes," you are not alone with these feelings.

Evaluation is something we all would rather not have. Someone cleverly said, "Criticism is like medicine. It's easy to give but difficult to take."

"For most of us, a strong effort of will is required to accept criticism of our job-related skills or capacities. It is a rare individual who sees such criticism as potentially helpful. More often we gripe about unfair or insensitive superiors and bemoan our inability to criticize them back. Or we grumble about coworkers who are always telling us what we are 'doing wrong' but never seem to listen to our complaints about their work."[1] But if we stop and think about it seriously, criticisms may be painful, but they are necessary.

Criticism provides a feedback from the people we work with

about how we are doing on the job site. This feedback becomes a "mirror" through which we can discover reflections of ourselves, whether good or bad. The feedback from our coworkers helps us to see the "blind spots" in our lives that our ego doesn't allow us to see.

Criticism also shows us things or areas we need to improve on and in this way, increase our output and our values to others in the workplace. It fulfills the same function as fever in the body—it is a symptom that tells us something is not right, and that something needs to be done to correct that problem. In other words, criticism serves as a warning, to bring about change for the better. If taken in the right context, criticism can encourage self-improvement.

Dr. Hendrie Weisinger and Norman M. Lobsenz, in their book *Nobody's Perfect,* tell us, "Criticism is just a four-letter word: GROW!" If we allow it to, criticism can be a means of helping us to grow, and in this way, become better nurses.

If you ask people to tell you what criticism means, "Chances are they would overwhelmingly characterize it as an opinion or observation that is destructive, humiliating, or hostile, the purpose of which is to find fault."[2]

Dr. Honor Whitney, a family therapist, tells us, "A constant stream of negative remarks—sarcasm, doubts, rebuffs, put-downs— cut emotional scars into even the sturdiest ego." She goes on to state, "Ultimately, negative statements seriously undermine the way people feel about themselves. The self-image, the inner sense of value as an individual, is weakened."

As nurses, we all know one or two of our coworkers who always seem to excel in giving destructive criticisms. It seems that every word that comes out of their mouths is a "put-down" or a blame for one thing or another. They seem to thrive on making others feel "small." They use their criticisms as sledgehammers or axes to cut others down. Somehow it seems like making others feel "small" makes them feel "big." In short, these people seem to always bring out the worst in us.

God, in His infinite wisdom, sometimes puts these "special" nurses in our lives in order to teach us patience and humility. In essence, they are blessings in disguise, and should be accepted as such. Let's praise God daily for sending them our way.

Our feelings usually run high when our yearly evaluations come around. First, salary increases depend on it. Secondly, peer evaluations play a major part in prospective promotions, and lastly, often our careers are greatly affected by a performance appraisal. It is imperative that we "look good."

Because our egos are fragile and because peer evaluations affect our careers, we have to be careful how we criticize. "As Christians, we have been given the responsibility to admonish—to criticize. But utmost caution must be used so that criticism benefits rather than damages, builds up rather than tears down, strengthens rather than weakens. We must be spiritual surgeons, not butchers."[3] We must be honest and fair, and care enough for the other person to want to bring about a change in their lives. People need to know that we really care for them when we criticize them.

Keep in mind these four examples of how not to evaluate:

1. Too lenient—evaluating everyone as outstanding so that their feelings aren't hurt. In other words, lying to make others feel good. Proverbs 28:23 informs us that people appreciate frankness rather than flattery.
2. Too strict—the opposite of being too lenient—rating everyone at the low end of the scale. It involves being too critical and demanding.
3. Too average—evaluating everyone as being average regardless of major differences in their performances.
4. Too subjective—basing your evaluation on subjective perceptions rather than objective facts. It is the tendency to rate a person based solely on an experience involving only one dimension. For instance, if your co-worker refuses to do something he was asked to do, and this incident is used against him three years later, and on every evaluation. It involves using personal opinions instead of facts.

When criticizing others, there are several things to take into consideration. First of all, is the criticism necessary? What do you want to teach the person you are criticizing? Have you prayed about this? Are you criticizing the person in the way that shows that you really care for him?

Here are some ideas for giving criticism:

1. Pray for that person and ask the Holy Spirit to reveal to you how to confront him.
2. Be sensitive about when and where to give the criticism. Remember that your objective is not to shame or embarrass the other person, but to teach him and bring about a change in his life.
3. Target the behavior that needs to be changed, and not the person.
4. Do not allow your own negative feelings of pride, anger and hostility to tint the criticism.
5. Offer ways to help the person to change the behavior.
6. If the person begins to show an improvement, remember to give verbal recognition and appreciation for that improvement, no matter how small it might be.

"Anyone who attempts to do anything worthwhile has to learn to take criticism, constructive or otherwise. And it is often those who accomplish the most in the long run who are pelted with the most criticism. Criticism is the price for accomplishment and adventure."[4] Even though it hurts, let us accept our criticisms and grow.

Prayer: My Heavenly Father, I don't like evaluations and criticism, but, Lord, I know they are supposed to make me grow, not only as a nurse, but also as a Christian. Help me to accept these and use them as steps to improve myself. And when I am in the position to evaluate others, let me remember that my objective is to build up and to bring about change, not to break down and destroy the other person. And Lord, remind me of the importance of letting people know how much they are appreciated when they excel at something, no matter how small it might be.

Thank You for Your love that makes me want to be a better Christian nurse. Amen.

Thought: Lord, when we are wrong, make us willing to change, and when we are right, make us easy to live with.
—Peter Marshall

Notes

1. Dr. Hendrie Weisinger and Norman M. Lobsenz, *Nobody's Perfect: How to Give Criticism and Get Results* (Los Angeles, CA: Warner Books, 1981), pp. 198–99.
2. Ibid., p. 4.
3. Lars Wilhelmsson, *Making Forever Friends* (Torrance, CA: Martin Press, 1982), p. 135.
4. Ibid., p. 141.

James 2:2–4—For if there come unto your assembly a man with a gold ring, in goodly apparel, and there come in also a poor man in vile raiment; and ye have respect to him that weareth the gay clothing, and say unto him, sit thou here in a good seat; and say to the poor, stand thou there, or sit here under my footstool: are ye not the partial in yourselves and are become judges of evil thoughts?

24
Favoritism

How do you react when the patient assigned to your care is dirty and filthy, with teeth that are rotten and yellow? He might look like a bum or a drunk from the rescue mission or skid row. He might be overweight and unattractive, and there might be a stench of urine and vomit about him. His skin color may be darker than yours, or his eyes slanted. He might have been diagnosed with AIDS, or he might be yelling insults at you. How do you react to him? Do you have feelings of repulsion and disgust? Are you indifferent to him, do you ignore him, speak harshly to him, or try to stay as far away from him as possible for fear of being contaminated?

Now, how do you react when your patient is a celebrity? What if he's a Denver Bronco, or an actor, or the mayor of the city? He might be a rich VIP with numerous titles after his name and he might be attractive and wearing expensive clothes. How do you react to this one? Do you indulge him, pay more attention to him, cater to his every whim, spend more time with him than with your other patients, and give him the very best care possible? If you treat the first man with less respect than the second man, you're practicing favoritism.

Favoritism may be one of the most prevalent sins among Christians today. It is so common that at times we don't even recognize it as sin. The book of James (2:1–4) tells us that it is indeed a deadly sin to discriminate in this way and, notice this, James was writing to people who called themselves Christians! Favoritism was a problem in the New Testament days, and it is still a problem among Christians today. There are other synonyms for favoritism: snobbery, prejudice, partiality, preferential treatment. No matter what you call it, the book of James regards this behavior as being unworthy of a true Christian. The Bible tells us that even God and Jesus hated favoritism (Acts 10:34).

"Is a jewel less precious because it comes in a plain box? Is a person less important when bound up with what we judge to be a limited mind or an unattractive outward appearance? As the Bible bluntly puts it, to show partiality or favoritism is not good (Proverbs 28:21)."[1] When we practice favoritism, it makes us judges over other people. We take the judgment from the hands of God (Who is the real Judge, and Who has the right to judge), and place it in our own hands. We make poor judges. We look on the outward appearance, which can be very deceiving. God is equipped to judge because He is flawless and no respecter of outward appearances. He alone looks into the heart of a person.

As Christian nurses, we should love, respect, and treat all our patients with dignity, regardless of their position in society, financial resources, or physical appearance. This is what Jesus Christ commands. Favoritism keeps people from knowing about Jesus Christ and about His saving grace. We are so busy trying to please people that we don't take the time to reach souls for Christ. Christ Jesus died for the poor, filthy soul as well as for the rich VIP soul, and all people need to know how much He cares for them. What Jesus Christ wants should matter to us as Christian caregivers, not what society expects or wants from us. We should strive to please Him because He is the One to whom we will eventually have to give an account of our lives. Let us remember, we are <u>all</u> made in God's image—<u>all</u> His children—<u>all</u> loved equally by Him.

Favoritism is wrong. It takes the glory away from our deserving God and gives it to man, who isn't worthy of it. We are glorifying the rich and powerful when we should be reserving that glory for Almighty God, alone.

We practice favoritism for selfish reasons. We want to make

people feel good, to make ourselves feel good, and to gain some favor in return. Our true inner motives may be to flatter others for our own advantages and our own selfish needs. God's glory doesn't even come into consideration. Selfish pride also plays a part in favoritism. Sometimes, we feel that we are superior to others, and this causes us to be partial only to those who fit into our own special categories for acceptability.

For a Christian to behave in this way is tragically wrong, and unbecoming a child of God. Below are guidelines for fighting favoritism:

1. Confess Your Sins: Of favoritism, discrimination, prejudice, and partiality, and ask Jesus Christ to give you a clean and pure heart to love others the way you should. Favoritism is sin, short and simple, and sin is breaking the laws God has laid down for us as Christians. It is violating the principles He has revealed to us which are important in the lives of His people. We as Christian nurses must strive to eradicate this kind of sin from our lives if we are going to become victorious and productive Christians in His service to our patients and their families. If we confess our sins, the Bible tells us God is faithful and just and will forgive our sins and cleanse us from all unrighteousness.

2. Practice Tolerance: Get to know people who are different—people of other races, religions, nationalities. Listen to them and find out what makes them tick. Humbly allow yourself to be taught about others with whom you may not be readily comfortable. Often our discomfort stems from the unknown—rather than any "perceived" wrong. Don't consider yourself better than they are because you may be cleaner, better educated, or make more money. Jesus Christ our Lord and Savior died for these people, too, and that makes them valuable to Him. In His eyes, you and I are no better than anyone else. He loves and cares for them just as much as He does for you and me. His life here on earth and His death on the cross attest to the love He has for all people, and this includes the skid row bum, the

AIDS victim, the vulgar drug addict, the black woman without health insurance, and the 500-pound man. Like you and me, they are also precious in His sight, and part of His handiwork.

3. <u>Learn to Love Others Unconditionally:</u> Our prejudice and favoritism cause us to reject those who are different, especially people we feel are "beneath" us. This is not biblical. We must accept and love people unconditionally. The Bible tells us in Matthew 11:19 that Jesus Himself is a "friend of tax collectors and sinners." We might not condone their sin, lifestyle, or their belief system, but like Jesus Christ, we must love them and accept them as people made in the image of God, and treat them with dignity and respect. We must love them regardless of their status, color, beliefs, and lifestyle, and love them <u>all</u> equally, the way Christ Jesus loves us all.

4. <u>Look at Others through the Eyes of Jesus:</u> When we look at others through the eyes of Jesus Christ, it is not so difficult to love them with all their faults and inadequacies. This makes it easy for us to look past the filthy clothes, repulsive breath, foul language, different skin color and hair texture, and their diseased condition, and see another human being, made in the image of God, dearly loved by Jesus Christ. As Joseph Parker puts it, "He whose eye is filled with Christ never sees what kind of coat a man has on." 1 Samuel 16:7b tells us, "For the Lord seeth not as man seeth; for man looketh on the outward appearance, but the Lord looketh on the heart."

Friends and colleagues, remember that we will be called to give an account of our lives one of these days. "We'd better get our minds off color, and off who is rich or poor, who can speak the most correct language, and get our minds on who is ready to go to heaven, who needs to be saved, what can I do for the Lord, and how can I further His work?"[2] Let us, as Christian caregivers, get busy going about our calling. We need to bring Jesus Christ to a world that is dying. God wants us to be a light to the world. This includes even those people we might consider "undesirable." Look around you today. Souls may be at stake. People are sick and dying for that special light that only those who are Spirit-filled can bring. Are you willing to be used by Him? Are you willing to look past people's shortcomings and see souls that need salvation through Jesus Christ? If you are, then let's get busy! There is so much out there to be done.

Prayer: Father, forgive me my sin of favoritism. Teach me to love those that are placed in my care, with the love You've taught me in Your Word. When I look at my patients let me see people with needs—physical, emotional and spiritual needs— and help me to meet those needs in the best way I can. Remind me daily that we are *all* made in Your image and that we are valuable to You. Thank You for loving me unconditionally. In Your precious Name. Amen.

Thought: Christ can give supernatural love, which enables you to love even those whom innately you could not love.
—Billy Graham

Notes

1. John Blanchard, *Truth for Life,* (Hertfordshire, England: Evangelical Press, 1986), p. 118.
2. Jean Sherrill, *God Answers Racist Christians* (Jacksonville, AR: United We Stand Holiness Movement, 1983), p. 55.

Proverbs 9:9—Give instruction to a wise man, and he will be yet wiser: teach a just man, and he will increase in learning.

25
Breaking In the New Person

I don't think I will ever forget November 13, 1987—the day I started working at Swedish Medical Center. I had been a nurse for about 11 years working in my country, Liberia, as a supervisor of the pediatric ward in the hospital I worked in. I had a master's degree in maternal-child nursing. I was 34 years old and thought I was reasonably confident in myself, but when I walked into the SMC parking lot that day, I felt insecure, uneasy and very scared. I remember trying to find my way in and out of corridors and elevators and finally locating the floor. To this day, I can still remember the nurse who showed me around and those nurses who said or didn't say hello to me. I can remember those who smiled, who came up and invited me to the lunchroom and who made me feel welcome. I remember which nurses went beyond their call of duty to give me support and encouragement. And I also remember which nurses ignored me, put me down and made me feel like a leper. More than ten years later, I still remember how stressful that day had been for me, and I believe that is why I have a special spot in my heart for the new nurse on her first day at work.

The "newcomer" could be the new graduate, fresh from school and waiting to take the state board exams or the RN "between jobs" or seeking a new job. The "newcomer" could also be the RN who had left nursing for a period of years and is now coming back, or nursing students coming to the workplace for clinical experiences. No matter which type he or she is, the "newcomer" goes through feelings similar to the ones I experienced my first day at work. They all need help to adjust easily and smoothly to the workplace.

There are usually three major groups of people involved in orientation for the newcomer:

1. Personnel Office or Human Resources
2. Head nurse, nurse manager, supervisor
3. Peer

The Personnel Office or Human Resources provides information about hospital policies, benefits, parking information, employee health, leave, security, and office for continuing education, among many other items. The head nurse, nurse manager or supervisor provides additional information about the worksite, probation period, duties, performance appraisal, overtime, schedules, what types of uniforms to wear on the job, safety, etc. There is a lot of information given by these two groups, but these two have their limits.

Even though these groups provide a mountain of information necessary for the new job, this is not nearly enough to prepare a nurse for the workplace, where the rubber really meets the road. Here is where the real "classroom" is, where the "nitty gritty" of nursing is. This is where the importance of the peer orientation comes in. In this time of transition, the other nurses can either make or break the newcomer. The newcomer goes through a time of insecurity, tension, stress and uneasiness, fear about the new job, uncertainty and common mistakes.

The feelings of insecurity, tension, stress and uneasiness often causes her to behave in such a way that makes others think she lacks self-confidence. If a person looks stupid, people will think she really is stupid. "Coworkers quickly size up any flaws in the new person. Often the new employee is not aware of the first impression he or she is making and unwittingly comes across as slower, less friendly, or less enthusiastic than he really is."[1]

Fear about the new job might cause her to ask questions like, "Am I capable?" "Will I remember everything I learned in school?" "Will my coworkers like or accept me?" "Will I make a fool of myself?" or "Will I meet their expectations?" There is also an uncertainty about where a certain equipment is or where the nurses' lounge, cafeteria, bathroom, best parking space, and exits are. Along with the fear and uncertainty come the common mistakes newcomers usually make.

Some common mistakes are an inability to take criticism, an unteachable spirit, stubbornness about listening, and reluctance to ask questions or seek explanation of a procedure for fear of appearing stupid. Another mistake is having an attitude of arrogance, being a "know-it-all" or "smart aleck," or making statements like, "We did it differently at my last job."

Someone once said, "Nurses eat their young." I know this may sound harsh, but sometimes it appears like that is what we do to a newcomer. We usually do one of three things. We might shun them by ignoring them, giving them the silent treatment, gossiping about them or making sarcastic remarks and making them feel unwelcome. Perhaps we tolerate them until they have time to prove themselves. Or we accept them and make them feel welcome in the fold by showing them around and giving them the ins and outs of the floor. Sometimes some of us will go through all three steps, first shunning, then tolerating, and finally accepting the newcomer.

There are several reasons why we tend to shun the newcomer. Often the newcomer is seen as a threat and we think that if we don't help her out, maybe she will fail and be "let go." Some people are preoccupied with their own problems and don't want to be involved. Some don't know how to teach, and are insecure about what they know, therefore, don't want to precept other nurses. Still there are other people who like to wait until the newcomer "proves" herself. The newcomer is a stranger who has to prove she is capable before being accepted into the clan.

The probation period (which usually lasts for three months) is a time for testing, and the workplace is the testing ground. During this time, the newcomer has to cope not only with the job or her peers; she also has to cope with the head nurse or nurse manager. "Is she getting good reports or not?" And the fact that her economic survival depends on whether she makes it okay during the probation period and gets the job, all add to the stress she is already going through. All these things make it imperative that we all help the newcomer to fit in the workplace. Below are some suggestions on how to assist the newcomer and make her transition smooth and productive.

1. Make her welcome. Greet her with a smile and ask how she likes the place so far. A few words of conversation are appropriate. Ask her about where she worked before, and let her know that this hospital is a great place to work.
2. Be sensitive. Remember that this must be a very stressful time for her. Give her a chance to prove herself—don't assume that she's stupid or a "space-cadet," just because she made a mistake or couldn't do a specific procedure. Remember that she's going through a learning process like we all are.
3. Introduce her to the workplace. Take her around and introduce her to the other nurses, ward clerks and doctors. Show her the bathrooms, exits, and other significant places. Also inform her about the different equipment used on the floor, and about special procedures. Advise her about things that are or aren't allowed on the floor. Each workplace has its own unique ways of doing things, and its own unique sets of rules. Teach her about what is accepted or not accepted on the floor.
4. Encourage and support her. Let her know that she can depend on you and that she should feel free to ask you for help. Teach her the right way if she's doing a procedure incorrectly, and praise her when she is doing fine.
5. Be patient with her. Remember, Rome wasn't built in one day. Be willing and open to learn from her—you'll be surprised how much knowledge she has herself.

These suggestions will help the newcomer to fit in and make the transition a rewarding and uplifting experience for her. In this way she will become a more productive nurse.

Prayer: Dear Lord, when I am in the position to precept others, help me to be patient, giving, and sensitive to their needs. Help me to assist them in every way to make their transition to the workplace smooth and productive. Remind me daily, that You put me here to uplift others, and that I am an ambassador for You. Thank You for calling me into the ministry. Amen.

Thought: The only difference between stumbling blocks and stepping stones is the way you use them.
—Author Unknown

Note

1. Nathaniel Stewart, *Winning Friends at Work: Your Relationships Can Be More Satisfying—Personally and Professionally* (New York: Ballantine Books, 1985), p. 117.

2 Thessalonians 3:10—For even when we were with you, this we commanded you, that if any would not work, neither should he eat.

26
Hard Work/Low Pay

There are many reasons why people work. Some have one reason, others more than one. Perhaps the most common reasons are for money and security.

There is the single mother who needs money to put bread on the table, and the mother and father who need two paychecks to support their family. Another is a woman who just got divorced and is now in charge of her own financial affairs. Then there's the nurse who is reentering the nursing profession after a period of staying home to care for the family, and now needs extra money. There is also the foreigner who has come to this country in order to break out of the circle of poverty. Then there is the nurse who just wants more money for luxury and the extra things in life.

Another reason why people work is not necessarily for the money, but for the feeling of personal progress. They work for the special benefits, to have an impressive résumé, to prove self-worth, or as a measure of recognition, respect and admiration. Being paid for something they enjoy doesn't hurt either. Others work because of the social values of work: to make friends, for companionship, acceptance, a sense of belonging, support, and having fun.

Lastly, some people work in order to lead a more purposeful life, to gain self-fulfillment, and self-realization. They believe that they have a purpose in life; therefore, they use their skills and knowledge to make contributions to society, or to a group of people. The Christian nurse who goes to a Third World country to minister to the poor and needy is an example of this type.

No matter what your reasons for working, they all lead to one conclusion: satisfying human needs. Josh McDowell (*Building Your Self-Image*) mentions three basic emotional needs common to all people: first, the need to feel loved and to have a sense of belonging; second, the need to feel acceptable or to have a sense of worthiness; and thirdly, the need to feel adequate or to have a sense of competence. Work fulfills all three of these needs and helps us better understand ourselves and others.

Job satisfaction is very important, and two essential factors for this satisfaction are peer relationships and salary. Peer relationships are vital for four major reasons: teamwork, confiding, learning, and fellowship.

Teamwork

The expression, "Two heads are better than one," is very true, or in this case, "Two or more heads are better than one." In teamwork we are partners for better or worse. We stand together and meet the physical, emotional and spiritual needs of our patients and their families. This involves a collaboration that must be nurtured and cultivated. It must involve mutual respect, trust, confidence, concern and love. We can't always choose who we work with but we have to at least <u>like</u> working with the others on the team.

"Genuine collaboration can help peers reach astonishing heights of performance. By merging talents and energies toward a common goal, working partners are able to produce results more effectively, on a timely basis, and with the kind of perspective that one person alone could hardly accomplish. They are able to pool experience and expertise to probe a [company] problem more deeply and to see more clearly the various alternatives in solving the problems."[1] Teamwork also provides a sense of personal satisfaction for everyone involved. Teamwork involves growing and learning together as partners.

Confiding

Confiding is more than just getting along with your peers. It involves sharing confidences—expressing pain, hurt, pride, joy and elation. We share our headaches, heartaches, lost loves, new loves, our son's award won in swimming, our daughter's new boyfriend, our Pap test results, our marriages, our divorces, and our pets.

People confide in others for several reasons: to share news about developments in their lives, to get help in solving problems they might have, to allow others to share in their joys and sadness, for sympathy and empathy, and to reinforce self-esteem.

Learning

There is no question that peer relationships involve learning from one another. Each nurse has skills and gifts unique to her, and we learn by tapping into these resources. It doesn't matter what floor or ward you work on, you will always find that some nurses are outstanding for their special gifts and skills.

There are those gifted in planning and organizing; it seems like they are always in control. They know where everything is or should be. They know how everything is run.

There are those who are great in doing certain procedures like starting IVs or drawing lab specimens, or tending very critical patients. They are a whiz in special areas of nursing. Then there are those who excel in leadership—they are General Patton in times of emergencies, and are at their very best when placed in charge of other nurses.

There are those nurses who love to give not only their money, but also their possessions and their time for other nurses. They uplift others with affirmation, encouragement, advice, by listening, by jokes and prayers. They seem to have contagious joy and happiness and when you are around them, you can't help smiling. Then there are those who are great teachers. Just give them a topic and stand back and watch them in action.

If you look around your workplace today you will find nurses who have these special qualities. Some have one, others several. God has equipped each of us with gifts and special skills; when we use those gifts and skills for the benefit of other nurses on the team, we receive the rich satisfaction that is experienced by those who give of what God has given them.

We can only learn from each other when we respect others' gifts and skills. The experiences of the seasoned veteran or the "old pro" who has been around for a while and knows the ropes, the expertise of the nurse who excels in certain areas, and the new ideas we learn from other nurses, all help us to learn things we don't get to learn in the classroom.

Fellowship

Fellowship in the workplace can be very helpful and fulfilling. These types of friendships, even though they sometimes last only the hours we work together, can be a source of satisfaction for everyone involved. Like any kind of friendship, the friendship we make at work needs to be cultivated and cared for. It takes effort, energy and time. It also involves respect, trust, loyalty, confidentiality, support and unconditional acceptance, among other qualities.

This kind of friendship is cultivated in a social setting and involves building a career together, using each other's skills and gifts, and earning a living together. It might last for only the four, six, eight or twelve hours we spend working with each other, or it can extend to time outside the workplace, when we go skiing, vacationing, dining out, watching a movie, or just visiting together.

It doesn't matter how much time we spend together or where we spend that time, friendship in the workplace meets and satisfies our human needs of love, acceptance, competence and worthiness. We need this type of friendship for job satisfaction.

The other factor that is essential for job satisfaction is salary. Working as nurses, we sometimes have to make significant sacrifices. Sometimes we have to give up valuable time we should be spending with family and loved ones, in order to work weekends, holidays and overtime. We also give up time we should be spending enjoying ourselves.

In addition to time, we also miss out on some material comforts. For example, while others are sleeping soundly in their warm beds on winter nights, we are awake on tired feet, turning patients, changing dressings, starting IVs, emptying bedpans, fluffing pillows, giving back rubs, and ministering to our patients and their families.

Some people believe that in addition to time and material comforts, nurses also lose out on the salary they should be making. Some individuals get depressed when they hear what people are making in real estate, pro sports, or as a doctor. They see other people who have Corvettes, and live in very expensive homes, while they still drive 1984 Toyotas and are still renting apartments.

I used to think that if I loved and enjoyed the job I was doing, compensation for my work as a nurse would be a minor issue. I have found out now that I was really wrong. Money problems and unpaid bills that keep piling up can take the joy out of our work.

"Making a lot of money is a bad reason, if it's the only reason, for choosing a vocation. In fact the chances of succeeding at making large sums of money in a profession are greatly reduced if you don't inherently love the work. But make no mistake, it is difficult—almost impossible—to love your work if you can't support yourself and your family, if you're constantly struggling to make ends meet, or if you have a chronic sense of being underpaid."[2] Let's face it, the bills come rolling in (on time) every month, but money doesn't.

Like it or not, a "good pay communicates worth."[3] A raise or increment in my salary indicates that I am of worth. The raise is an affirmation of what the people I work for think of me. The better I am at my job, the more money I make. Problems arise when we feel that even though we are working very hard at our jobs, we are still being underpaid. This feeling usually comes about when we compare our salaries with other professions. For example, most of us believe that athletes are paid too much money for just playing ball or that actors are paid too much for just acting, while nurses work harder and longer, and get paid a lot less.

We also tend to compare our salaries with those of other nurses. Some questions we ask are: "How come she makes more than I do? She's just a diploma nurse." Or, "We do the same job, how come she makes more than I do?"

In our quest to make big bucks, we tend to look at other people's wealth with envy instead of being grateful for what we have and doing the best with it. There are so many nurses in other countries around the world who don't make even one-third of what nurses make here in America, but who are able to meet the needs of their families, because they have learned to rely on God for meeting their needs.

J. Hudson Taylor puts it simply, "Depend upon it, God's work done in God's way will never lack God's supplies." We have been called to God's service. He will surely provide for us. Paul tells us in Philippians 4:19, "But my God shall supply all your needs according to his riches in glory by Christ Jesus." God will supply all my needs. The Bible says it and I believe it.

Sometimes the problem isn't what we make, but what we do with the money that we get. God wants us to have good things and to enjoy them. He also wants us to use the money He has given us in a prudent manner. At times we misuse the money and then wonder why we can't pay our bills on time.

Paul admonishes us in Philippians 4:11 to be contented in whatsoever state we are in. And 1 Timothy 6:6–8 states, "But godliness with contentment is great gain. For we brought nothing into this world, and it is certain we can carry nothing out. And having food and raiment let us be therewith content." My friends, let us be contented with what we already have, and let us be careful how we spend the wealth that God has blessed us with.

Prayer: God, thank You for the job You have provided for me. Thank You also for the people You have placed in my workplace. May I learn and grow with them. My Heavenly Father, You hold the wealth of all creation in Your hands, and You can supply all my needs. Help me to remember

that the next time I start to envy other people's wealth. Thank You for everything You've given me. Amen.

Thought: Contentment is natural wealth; luxury, artificial poverty.

—Socrates

Notes

1. Nathaniel Stewart, *Winning Friends at Work: Your Relationships at Work Can Be More Satisfying—Personally and Professionally* (New York: Ballantine Books, 1985), p. 73.
2. Janis Long Harris, *Secrets of People Who Love Their Work* (Downers Grove, IL: Intervarsity Press, 1992), p. 103.
3. Ibid., p. 96.

1 Corinthians 15:55—O death, where is thy sting? O grave, where is thy victory?

27
Death and Dying

Death is a subject no one likes to talk about. It seems too morbid. But death and dying are things we will come in contact with sooner or later in our career. There are some important things to understand about death.

First, the Bible tells us that everyone will die, no one is exempted. In the Book of Genesis, when Adam and Eve were tempted by Satan to disobey God, their sin brought the penalty of death to the whole human race. Because of their sin, we all will die someday.

Secondly, no one can cheat death. We all want to live on forever. The trend toward good and healthy living, eating properly, and exercising attest to this. But when the time comes (and it will), there will be nothing to do but go.

Finally, there is life after death. Not reincarnation into an animal, like some people believe, but eternal life with Christ Jesus—or without Him.

What is death? "Idealists have called it 'an illusion,' and romanticists speak of it as 'man's last great venture.' Poets have referred to it as 'crossing the river' and 'putting out to sea.' Atheists say that it is the end of existence. But all such concepts are empty and offer no hope."[1] Our definition of death depends greatly on our expectations from life. "Our expectations shape our behavior, beliefs and values. What we expect life to be, and the meaning we attach to the ending of that life, define what dying means to us."[2] Dying may mean different things to different people. It may mean a loss, a change, suffering, fear of the unknown, or a triumph.

A Loss

Death means a separation from people we love and from people who love us and need us. It separates us from places and things we treasure and from things we will no longer be able to do or be here on earth. It robs us of the opportunity of using the gifts and capacities God has given us. This loss can be painful.

A Change

Death brings about change (which can be an unwanted change). For some, death means having to live alone in a big house that had been occupied with a lifelong mate, for others it means having to live without a parent or a child, and still for others, it means having to take over being the sole support for the family. Death brings about changes that might involve leaving our comfort zone and venturing into the unknown.

Suffering

Death may mean suffering which can come in the form of pain, loneliness, or guilt. Death destroys the body first, breaking it down, creating mental confusion, total helplessness, and dependence upon others.

Fear of the Unknown

Death does have an aura of mystery around it that makes people afraid of it. We are leaving a life we are familiar with for one that is unfamiliar, and this can be very scary. This fear is like the fear that comes about when we venture to do something we've never done before. It carries the uncertainty of doing something new.

A Triumph

Death can also mean a triumph, especially for Christians. As nurses, some of us have cared for patients who seem to welcome death with a strength and peace that others don't have. John Metzger was one of those patients in my care. He had been living for years with ulcers, but you couldn't tell how much he was suffering by being around him. He was always smiling, and his sense of humor, joy, and tranquility in the midst of a terrible illness was truly amazing to see. He seemed to have no fear of death. To him, death meant being in the presence of Jesus Christ—a sort of homecoming. It was a strange and beautiful feeling. A few years later, when John died, I was privileged to be at his funeral, and it was a real homecoming. In that church that day, the verse that kept coming to my mind was: "O death, where is thy sting? O grave, where is thy victory?"

Death for a born-again Christian brings hope beyond the grave (Proverbs 14:32). It means permanent freedom from evil, hatred, envy, and greed. It means freedom from pain, sickness, suffering and strife. It means rest from life's toils and hardships, from bills and taxes. Most importantly, it means that we will see Christ Jesus face to face! Because of these things, Christians like John Metzger can smile and laugh in the face of death and be optimistic—something people who don't know God cannot understand.

The Bible tells us we are strangers on this earth. Our home is on the "other side" (2 Corinthians 5:1). As the songwriter states, "This world is not my home, I'm just a-passing through." The Word tells us our citizenship is in heaven, and when we die, we are going home where we belong, where there will be no more pain, suffering, sin, and, yes—no more death. The fear of death is removed. There is hope beyond death and that hope is centered in the risen Christ. Without Him and His death on the cross, there would be no hope (Proverbs 14:32). His death and His resurrection took away the sting of death. God offers this eternal life to everyone, regardless of race, sex, or creed. He offers it to whoever puts his trust and faith in Christ Jesus.

To a Christian, there are two kinds of death: a physical death and a spiritual death. A physical death, according to the Bible, is a separation of the soul from the body. This soul leaves the body and what is left is an empty shell (which is placed in the grave). The soul is not buried, but goes instead somewhere else. This means that physical death is not the end. The Bible teaches that the end of one (the physical death) is the beginning of another (the spiritual death), which is just as real as the last.

Revelation 20:14 tells us about the second death, which has to do with the state of a person's soul after the physical death. For believers in Christ, this physical death is wonderful news, but for nonbelievers, it means something terrible—a separation from God, or a spiritual death. "For the one who has not received Christ as Saviour, then, physical death—separation of the soul from the body—is but the portent of a far more dreadful aspect of death; it is the eternal separation of the soul from God."[3] Revelation 20:15 informs us that nonbelievers will be cast into the lake of fire. What a scary thought! In that lake of fire, there will be no "Rest-In-Peace." Only those who die in Christ will find rest from their labors after their physical death (Revelation 14:13).

If all it takes for a person to escape this terrible and dreadful end in the lake of fire is to become a believer, how come so many people are choosing to go to the lake of fire? How come we as Christian nurses are not hard at work, trying to help reduce the amount of people going toward the lake of fire, instead of toward eternal life with Jesus Christ? And why are we more concerned with the physical death and not the spiritual death which means eternal damnation in the lake of fire?

Caring for the Terminally Ill

A terminal illness is one from which recovery is beyond reasonable expectation. The illness may be the result of an accident, injury, or due to a disease condition. It is important to remember, however, that there have been many cases where doctors and nurses have given up hope for a patient who has subsequently been miraculously healed and has recovered entirely.

Our Heavenly Father, the greatest Physician of them all, is still in the business of healing people. There are good reasons, especially for us as Christian nurses, to retain hope when caring for terminally ill patients. It is also important for us as caregivers to understand how patients respond to the knowledge of imminent death in order for us to better meet their special needs. Understanding the patient's attitudes and feeling about death and dying makes us better prepared to deal with those feelings and attitudes when we do encounter them in our patients.

According to Dr. Elisabeth Kübler-Ross, a psychiatrist who specializes in counseling the terminally ill and their families, the terminally ill person passes through five emotional stages when told the end is near. They are: denial, resentment/anger, bargaining, depression, and finally, acceptance. These stages do not always follow one another. Sometimes they overlap, and their duration may vary from person to person. Even Christians go through these feelings.

The initial response, denial, leads the patient to refuse to believe that death is imminent. The patient might express his denial by saying, "No, there must be a mistake. It's not going to happen to me. God won't let it happen." During the next stage of anger/ resentment, his reaction is generally, "Why me?" In this stage, his anger may be directed at God, friends and family, and at those caring for him. When he proceeds to the bargaining stage, he begins to barter with God for an extension of life, and at this time, he might be receptive to the Word of God. The depression stage is indicated by an acknowledgement of impending death. The patient often experiences feelings of loneliness and depression until the final stage of acceptance. Here, the patient is able to say, "I'm ready to go."

"This term [acceptance] used by Dr. Kübler-Ross doesn't adequately indicate the difference between the attitude of the nonbeliever toward his death and that of the mature, yielded Christian. It's one thing to submit to the unavoidable, but it's quite another to be joyful in anticipation."[4] For the believer, it's a time to go from acceptance to joyous expectation because he is convinced that beyond death is the hope of eternal life. Our patients need to know that this kind of hope is available for anyone, in Jesus Christ.

What can we do as Christian caregivers to help our patients who are dying? Below are some guidelines for reaching out to those patients:

1. Evaluate your own feelings about death and dying. Work through your own inner conflicts about what you would do if you were told you didn't have long to live.
2. Listen with your heart to patients and their families who are dealing with death and dying. Use silence, and good listening techniques.
3. Allow your patients and their families to express their emotions and feelings about what is taking place in their lives. We must allow them to vent those feelings. It is difficult to open ourselves to others' sufferings, especially if those people are our patients. David Glen (*Living and Dying*) describes what he calls "Surrogate Suffering Syndrome." This is when we don't let others work through their own feelings of hurt or loss. We want to shield them, but in essence we are trying to shield our own feelings. Allow them to cry, if they want to.
4. Be available and present as much as possible and be willing to offer whatever assistance you can to the patient and the family. Give them a shoulder to lean on, cry on, or just hold on to.
5. Support and respect the patient and help him to maintain self-identity and his sense of worth in the midst of this terrible illness.
6. Meet the physical needs of the patients and their families to the best of your ability.
7. Pray for them, and with them, if they are open to that. Let them know you are available to pray with them.
8. Tell them about Jesus Christ (see chapter 39 on witnessing to the patients). Let them know how to accept Him, and tell them what happens when a person gives his life to Him. Let them know that when they accept

Jesus Christ as Lord and Savior, at the time of death they will change this frail and sick body for one that will never die or deteriorate, and be in a place where pain, suffering, disease and death can no longer touch them or harm them. Introduce them to Jesus Christ who has already defeated death, and do it right away, before it is too late!

Prayer: Jesus, thank You for the assurance that because You took my place at the cross and shed Your precious blood for my sins, today I am guaranteed eternal life. I know that physical death is not the end and that people need to know that. Let me be concerned enough about people in my care to point them toward You, so that they too can have that guarantee. Amen.

Thought: Oh, how we need to remind ourselves of the hope we have in Christ. When called upon to say that last goodbye to a Christian loved one, we can be comforted in knowing that for the departed this separation marks the last of earth's sorrows and the beginning of heaven's joys.

—Dennis J. DeHaan

Notes

1. Herbert Vander Lugt, *Light in the Valley: A Christian View of Death and Dying* (Wheaton, IL: Victor Books, 1979), p. 9.
2. Glen W. Davidson, *Living with Dying* (Minneapolis, MN: Augsburg Publishing House, 1975), p. 16.
3. Vander Lugt, *Light in the Valley,* p. 13.
4. Ibid., p. 28.

Part Four

Things We Need More Of

As she goes about her ministry, the Christian nurse needs special tools that will enable her to be the best she can be. This section offers ideas, suggestions and advice on how to obtain and maintain these valuable tools.

> 1 Peter 3:14–15—But and if ye suffer for righteousness' sake, happy are ye: and be not afraid of their terror, neither be troubled; But sanctify the Lord God in your hearts: and be ready always to give an answer to every man that asketh you a reason of the hope that is in you with meekness and fear.

Galatians 5:22–23—But the fruit of the Spirit is love, joy, peace, long-suffering, gentleness, goodness, faith, Meekness, temperance: against such there is no law.

28
Fruits of the Spirit

For the past ten years, my friend Anna has planted a garden on an acre of land at a community garden center. Each spring she carefully prepares the ground and removes leaves, rocks and other debris from the soil, making the ground soft and accessible for the seeds. Then she plants the precious seeds into the soil, being careful to plant them deep enough so that they can take root. But her work is not finished yet. Now she must make sure the seed grows properly; so she waters, weeds and prunes the garden, and waits patiently in anticipation for the seeds she has planted to grow and to produce.

As she waits, she enjoys watching the bees as they busily move from plant to plant, pollinating flowers, and the ladybugs, butterflies and hummingbirds that bring such beauty to her little garden. Finally comes the day of harvest when the fruits of her garden are available for consumption, and she gathers red, juicy tomatoes, big, leafy greens, plump zucchinis and cucumbers, golden ears of sweet corn, and other vegetables.

The fruit is what Anna and other gardeners and farmers anticipate when they plant a seed. The fruit is evidence of life. Likewise, the fruits of the Spirit give evidence of life in the Christian believer.

The fruits of the Spirit are those qualities people will remember you by if you call yourself a spiritually fit Christian. The book of Galatians, 5:22 and 23 lists the fruits of the Spirit. They are: love, joy, peace, long-suffering, gentleness, goodness, faith, meekness and temperance.

Love

We are required to love not only God, but also all people. This quality describes vividly the very nature of God Himself (1 John 4:8). This is the type of self-sacrificing love that brought our Lord Jesus Christ down to earth to die in our place (John 3:16). The book of 1st Corinthians, chapter 13, describes love in a simple and understanding way.

Joy

Joy is described as a constant delight and elation in God, and a cheerfulness in conversation. This is more than mere happiness, which usually depends on circumstances. Joy is related to our abiding in Christ Jesus, and allowing Him to abide in us (John 15:7–11).

Peace

This fruit is the opposite of worry and anxiety. It comes about when you turn your burdens over to Jesus Christ, refuse to worry, and rest in Him (Philippians 4:6–7). This requires the complete control of the Holy Spirit in our lives. It cannot be bought or inherited; Jesus Christ gives it freely. All we have to do is accept it. Of course, this acceptance depends upon our accepting Him as our Lord and Savior.

Long-suffering

This fruit is sometimes referred to as patience, and it means that you are able to put up with people who are simply difficult to work or live with. It also means to defer anger when your normal reaction would be to lash out in an outburst of anger, or to bear pain, trials, injuries and unpleasantness, without complaint.

David Hocking best describes long-suffering as, "taking a long time to boil."

Gentleness

Gentleness refers to a sweetness of disposition or temper, especially when others deliberately and spitefully wrong you. It keeps a person from trying to seek revenge or to inflict punishment upon those who have degraded or hurt him or his loved ones.

Goodness

Goodness or kindness is a desire to work for the good and benefit of another person, even when that person is unresponsive or undeserving of that kindness. It involves seeking to lift the burdens off the shoulders of others, and a readiness to do good to all people as we find the opportunities to do so.

Faith

Faith is connected with hope and is characterized by a constant dependency upon God. The Bible tells us that without faith, it is impossible to please God (Hebrews 11:6). It implies putting your confidence entirely in God and His abilities.

Meekness

Meekness means to govern our passions and resentments towards others, so as not to be easily provoked, and when we are provoked, to be soon pacified. Some confuse meekness with a weakness in character, or being a coward. This is far from the truth. It takes real strength to stand there and take it, when you are confronted with hostility and hatred, especially when you didn't deserve it in the first place. Jesus Christ gave an excellent example of meekness. As He was led away to be crucified, He was as meek as a lamb led to slaughter. He had multitudes of holy angels at His disposal, and He could have easily done something to save Himself, yet He stood there in meekness and took it all because He truly loved us. The most incredible thing is, when He left heaven, He knew He was coming to the cross to die for our sins! Nothing could stop Him from fulfilling the gospel, so He stood there—in our place. He is the best example of meekness. The Bible also tells us the meek shall inherit the earth (Matthew 5:5).

Temperance

Temperance or self-control is a virtue of a person who has a control over his or her passions and desires. It often applies to sexual appetites, but also applies to physical appetites like desire for food and drink. It is not easy to be self-controlled in these areas and we need the help of the Holy Spirit in order to be victorious over these appetites and habits.

These nine fruits have certain qualities. First of all, they are visible. People will look for these in those of us who profess to be Christians. They will see the love, joy, peace, long-suffering, gentleness, goodness, faith, meekness and temperance in our lives, and know that we are different from other people, because of our unique relationship with Jesus Christ.

Another quality of the fruits is that they are attractive. Do you remember the last time you went shopping for groceries? Did you notice how attractive the fruits and vegetables looked? The apples are spread out in different shades of red, yellow and green; the oranges, grapefruits, and tangerines look succulent, the plums, pears and grapes appear scrumptious and tempting. These fruits and vegetables attract you to them. The storekeepers keep their skins smooth and beautiful, not old and shriveled, because they want you to like them enough to pick them up and place them in your shopping baskets. In the same way, a Christian who is filled with the fruits of the Holy Spirit is a beautiful person not just to look at, but also to live with and to work with. People will inspect you daily for these qualities.

The fruits also attract unbelievers. They bring about a change in your life—a change for the better. Others (especially unbelievers) will see these changes in you and desire to experience them also. So many people have come to know the Lord Jesus as their Savior because they have seen those changes in certain Christians whom they live or work with. Lastly, these qualities produce seeds for the next season. Because they are visible and attractive and because they bring people to the Lord, these unbelievers then accept Him, and the Holy Spirit comes to dwell in them and begins to plant those seeds which will bear fruits for the "next season" of crops. In this way we multiply, and others come to know the Lord. Being fruitful in the spiritual way is the result of a right relationship with Jesus Christ, and having a right relationship with Him involves a direct and constant obedience to His Word. There can be nothing less.

It is very important for us as Christian nurses to have these fruits of the Spirit because they will help us to lead not only our families and colleagues to Jesus Christ, but also our patients and their families. These fruits will bear witness of our faith.

As I researched this topic, I came to the realization that there were several of these qualities lacking in my own spiritual life. It is my prayer that the Holy Spirit will continue to manifest Himself in my life, so that I can begin to exhibit these qualities. I hope this is also your prayer today. There is so much to be done to bring lost souls to Jesus Christ. And be reminded, people will be inspecting us daily for these fruits of the Spirit.

Prayer: My Lord and Savior, there are still areas in my life that need to come under Your complete control and authority. Today I turn these areas over to You. Fill me with the fruits of Your Spirit, so that people around me will be attracted to You through me. Help me to live what I preach. Remind me daily that I am living a sermon every day of my life, and that these sermons are sometimes more effective than the sermons I preach. When I am in-

spected, let people see in me love, joy, peace, long- suffering, gentleness, goodness, faith, meekness and temperance. Amen.

Thought: The serene, silent beauty of a holy life is the most powerful influence in the world, next to the might of the Spirit of God.

—Blaise Pascal

1 John 4:7–8—Beloved, let us love one another: for love is of God; and everyone that loveth is born of God, and knoweth God. He that loveth not knoweth not God; for God is love.

29
Love

All through the centuries, poets, songwriters, singers, authors and philosophers have written, sung and talked about love. Someone once said that more poems have been written about it than any other topic. Romance books and magazines speak about falling in love, while the blues relate the pain that comes about when a person falls out of love. More and more speakers are telling us how to fall in love and stay in love, and the psychiatrists' offices are full of people who feel no one loves them.

Everyone speaks about how important love is, and how everyone should love others, yet love is one of those concepts that is often misused, misunderstood and carelessly tossed around. People say, "I love my dog," "I love asparagus," "I love you to death," or "I love to ski." What exactly is this thing called love?

The book of 1st Corinthians, chapter 13, gives us characteristics of love. This passage tells us what love is and is not. It states: love is patient, kind, searches for the truth, holds up under pressure, always believes the best about others, looks to the future rather than the past, and is always consistent. The passage goes on to state that love is not jealous, does not boast or embarrass others, is not arrogant or selfish, does not bring to mind wrongs suffered, and does not get angry easily. Seems like a tall order, doesn't it?

The Greek language has three words that describe the different dimensions of love. They are: *agape, philia* and *eros*.

Agape

Agape means a higher kind of love or a Godly love. This is the type of love God has for us—the type of love that made Him sacrifice His one and only Son for the sins of the world (John 3:16). This is also the type of love God expects us as Christians to have for Him and for others, a love that no one, in his own strength and by his own effort, could possibly have.

Agape is an unselfish, unconditional and sacrificial kind of love. It puts God and the well-being of others ahead of our own feelings. God expects us to have this type of love for every human being regardless of sex, race, denomination, position or possessions. *Agape* love does not discriminate. It welcomes all people, even those who don't fit in our neat little "circle." We are to love others as Christ loves us (John 15:12). His love is to be the standard of our love for others, even our enemies.

Christ's love for us was apparent when He agreed to leave heaven, and to come down to earth, to give His precious blood for our sins. That took genuine love. He continues to reveal that love for us to this very day.

How many of us would volunteer to give our lives for our friends?

Agape love lets others know that we are indeed born-again Christians. Incidentally, it is the first of the fruits of the Spirit, and should be the basis or foundation for all other relationships. It is placed first on the list of fruits for a very good reason.

1 Corinthians 13:1–3 tells us that even if we speak with tongues of men and angels, have the gift of prophecy, understand all mysteries and all knowledge, have enough faith to even move mountains, give all our belongings to feed the poor or even give our bodies to be burned—if we don't love others, we are nothing. We can be the best nurses, teachers, counselors, pastors, choir members or lay ministers—without love, we are nothing. Our love is what will convince others (especially those who don't know Jesus Christ personally) that we are truly born-again Christians.

Philia

Philia love is sometimes referred to as brotherly love or affection. It is the compassionate love we have for good friends, our parents and children. It is having a fondness or liking for someone else.

Do you know that the name Philadelphia comes from this root word *philia* and means "City of Brotherly Love"?

While *agape* love is inclusive and does not discriminate, *philia* love is more exclusive and reserved for people we are familiar with and whom we like to be with and do things with. This type of love is not for everyone. It is limited to a group of people we like and are fond of. *Philia* love works better if its foundation is *agape* love. "By itself, *philia* is a quiet, comfortable feeling for people we usually take for granted."[1]

Eros

Eros, the third dimension of love, is not mentioned anywhere in the Bible. It is a self-gratifying and passionate type that is the physical expression of love. It is self-centered, and short-lived passion seeking satisfaction that should be reserved for only one person, your spouse. Unfortunately, people misuse this type of love by utilizing it outside of marriage, thus leading to various kinds of problems for everyone involved. Most of the time *eros* does not have the *agape* and *philia* foundations and as soon as the erotic feelings decline, the individual starts to look somewhere else for that gratification. This type is more lust than love.

Billy Graham used this diagram to explain these three dimensions of love:

Eros (reserved for one person, your spouse)

Philia (limited to people you are fond of)

Agape (broad base—includes all people)

Foundation

With *agape* as a foundation, this relationship has the capacity to survive the "storms" of life when they come. More than often, people turn the triangle upside down making *eros* the foundation for their relationships, and even when a small "storm" comes, the relationship topples over because it doesn't have a firm foundation.

This brings me to the question: Why do we love or why should we love?

We love because Christ first loved us (1 John 4:19). About the measure of His love toward us, there is no question. Jesus Christ truly loves us. He portrayed that love for us when he came to die in our place, "that we might live through Him" (1 John 4:9). He did this despite our constant unfaithfulness and despite our repeated sins. The Bible tells us that "while we were yet sinners, Christ died for us" (Romans 5:8). And He loves us even though so many people still refuse to accept His gift of genuine love. "Beloved if God so loved us, we ought also to love one another" (1 John 4:11). When we love others, what we are doing is returning God's love.

We love because Jesus commands us to love others. John 15:12 tells us that Jesus said, "This is my commandment, that ye love one another, as I have loved you." This statement doesn't give alternatives; this is a direct order from our Lord and Savior. We must love others if we want to obey His commands. He is our example of love itself. His selfless love sets a standard for our love for others. God created us to love. In fact, He is love (1 John 4:8). He is the very essence of love (remember, we are made in His image); therefore, if we say He (the Holy Spirit) lives in us, we must love others.

We also love because others need our love. Within us all is the fundamental need to feel loved. According to Dr. Erich Fromm, loneliness and the inability to love are the underlying causes of emotional illness. "The fields of medicine and psychology agree that the overwhelming need of all people is love. People need to receive and give love. Love is the single most important force in shaping our lives. People either love or perish."[2] Love gives us the sense of belonging—a sense that is essential to our self-worth. We need to love and be loved.

People will know we are Christians by our love. Jesus said: "By this shall all men know ye are my disciples, if ye have love one to another" (John 13:35). We cannot reach others for Jesus Christ unless we have love in our hearts for them. Love will sensitize our hearts to the spiritual, emotional and physical needs of others. We cannot bring people to Christ by being judgmental; we can bring people to Him by our love. God gives love <u>to</u> us and <u>through</u> us. His love should flow through us to others. In our service to others, love must be our number one priority.

Love gives purpose to life. It restores marriages, heals broken hearts and homes, and unites families. It overcomes petty hatred, prejudice, resentment and bitterness. It defuses anger and conquers depression. It makes it easier to forgive people who have willfully wronged you. Love is our strongest weapon against Satan. It is God's gift to us and through us to those around us. We must be the channels of His love to the world.

Look around you today—the world is literally starving for love. Americans are people who give generously. When there is news of famine in Africa or drought in other parts of the world, Americans give money, food and medical supplies to help the starving people. Pictures of children with sunken eyes and bloated abdomens, with multitudes of flies invading their faces, tug at the hearts of every decent person and make them want to reach out to these needy people and support them financially.

But did you know that there is drought and famine right here in America? Yes, spiritual and emotional famine! There are people with broken lives, who need your spiritual and emotional support. And it doesn't cost you a thing. They need love. We all need love, and when we give love, we receive love in return.

I urge you today to reach out to people and let them know you love them. Be reminded that love can only be expressed through action. The things we say or do must relay to others that we truly love and care for them. As Christians we must take the first step in putting our love into action. Remember, they will know we are born-again Christians by our love. Our prayer should be as Dr. Will Houghton fittingly puts it:

Love this world through me, Lord
This world of broken men
Thou didst love through death Lord
Oh, love in me again!
Souls are in despair, Lord
Oh, make me know and care;
When my life they see, may they behold Thee,
Oh, love the world through me.

Prayer: My Heavenly Father, thank You for giving me the greatest gift of all—the gift of Your Son Jesus Christ, the ultimate gift of love. Jesus, fill me with Your genuine and perfect love, and channel that love through me to a world that is in dire need of love. Send someone my way today that I might relay that love. Thank You, Holy Spirit, for coming to live in me and for teaching me the meaning of genuine love. Amen.

Thought: God will one day ask us not about our confessions of faith, nor about our denominational membership. He will ask us, solely about love; what of His love could flow through us, and what of His love—that is of His being—took on form in us.

—Wilhard Becker

Notes

1. George Sweeting, *Love Is the Greatest* (Chicago, IL: Moody Press, 1974), p. 27.
2. Lars Wilhelmsson, *Making Forever Friends* (Torrance, CA: Martin Press, 1982), p. 38.

Isaiah 51:11—Therefore the redeemed of the Lord shall return, and come with singing unto Zion; and everlasting joy shall be upon their head: they shall obtain gladness and joy; and sorrow and mourning shall flee away.

30
Joy

Joy is one of the fruits of the Spirit. It is the second of these fruits and, next to love, is one of the most important ways people can tell that we are born-again Christians.

Just being a Christian doesn't bring joy. Unfortunately, some of the most unhappy people I know are Christians! Too often they walk around unhappy, gloomy and very miserable, living lives of defeat and negativity. They do not act as children of the King. They do not act like people who have been forgiven, saved and are on their way to heaven.

Vance Havner has said: "The average Sunday morning congregation appears as if it has gathered to mourn a defeat rather than celebrate a victory. Too many seem to be enduring their salvation instead of enjoying it. We need to remind ourselves that we've not been called to a funeral, but to a feast!" Too many people make it look like Christianity is only for people who don't want to have fun or to be happy. No wonder so many don't want to become Christians for fear that this would mean removing happiness and joy from their lives. No wonder they don't take Jesus Christ seriously!

Happiness is not the same as joy. Happiness depends on what happens to you. For example, a raise, a newborn or a new car might make you happy, but joy is independent of circumstances. "Happiness is like the surface of the sea—ever changing. Joy is like the ocean bed—ever the same."[1] It is impossible to be happy all the time, but joy can still abide despite what is happening in your life, because as Christians we know that our Heavenly Father will never leave us or forsake us, no matter what happens. Through hills and dales, through mountains and valleys, we have the assurance of the presence of His love, care and support in our lives. This assurance brings "unspeakable" joy to the life of the spirit-filled Christian.

Everyone wants to be happy and joyous, and some think they can find joy in fame, fortune or pleasure. Many think "if only I had enough money to buy a house with a swimming pool and a sauna, a Porsche, and a yacht, or if I could be able to travel the world, I would be happy!" Very soon, they find out that money doesn't necessarily bring them joy or happiness—in fact, it sometimes creates more problems.

Ernest Hemingway (the renowned author) had won both the Pulitzer and Nobel prizes, was very rich and famous, had expensive and exotic homes all over the world, and was described as a man with a "lust for life," who was "the life of the party." Yet in 1961, he put a gun to his head and ended his life. All his money, fame and popularity could not fill the emptiness inside.

Beauty, professional success or riches do not bring inner peace or joy either. Marilyn Monroe had all of these things and more, yet one day, she too ended it all by overdosing on pills. Those material objects could not satisfy her or give her inner peace or joy.

Others think power or position can give them joy. They would say, "If only I had that job or that promotion, I would be happy." But instead of joy, power brings with it disappointments, burnout, loneliness and suspicion.

Still others believe that they can achieve joy and happiness from alcohol and other drugs, which might elate a person, or elevate the mood for a while. The "joy" these give do not last. They bring about a sort of counterfeit joy, and afterwards, the person feels terrible, miserable and sick. Some people believe alcohol gives them courage and boldness—to say or do things they would not normally say or do. Of course, alcohol gives them a fake sense of courage and boldness that often gets them into trouble.

Certainly, the alcohol and other drugs give a "high," but there is no "high" without a "low." Eventually you have to come down and the "low" is even worse than before. You will keep needing more and more "highs."

There is no question about it—a person cannot achieve joy from fame, beauty, power, position, riches, success, alcohol or other drugs. "Trying to find satisfaction in the things of this world is like chasing soap bubbles, or trying to reach the pot of gold at the end of a rainbow."[2]

How then can a person find joy? Below are some suggestions:

In Jesus Christ

This involves accepting Him and having a personal relationship with Him. When you accept Jesus Christ, the Holy Spirit comes to live in your heart, and brings joy, the second fruit of the Spirit. The fruit of joy grows and flourishes when we are in obedience with His laws. Without Jesus Christ, you cannot have that "unspeakable" joy that is so essential in the Christian's life.

Prayer and Meditation in the Word

The Prophet Jeremiah stated in Jeremiah 15:16, "Thy words were found, and I did eat them; and thy word was unto me the joy and rejoicing of mine heart: for I am called by thy name, O Lord God of hosts." Truly the Word of God has within it ever-flowing fountains of joy. We must go daily to the Lord to maintain that feeling of elation and joy that come about when we are in a right relationship with the Lord. Our personal time with the Lord increases joy in our lives.

Praise, Worship and Fellowship with other Christians

Psalm 122:1 states, "I was glad when they said unto me, Let us go into the house of the Lord." How wonderful it is when you are among a group of people who truly love the Lord, praising, worshiping and fellowshipping together in His presence! It brings about a type of joy that is uplifting and contagious. Praising the Lord, especially with other believers, always brings joy.

Other Tools of Joy

There are other tools that help us maintain joy. Music is one of these tools. Years ago, as slaves labored in the hot southern sun, they kept up their spirits with song. In the midst of some of the worst times of degradation, poverty, hatred, and being treated as less than human beings, they sang joyful songs. People looked at them, and wondered, "How can they smile, sing and be happy at times like these?" Their love for the Lord made them sing despite the hardships they were going through. Some of the best Negro spirituals came about during this era.

The power of music lifts the heart above pain, degradation, humiliation and disappointments. It makes life bearable and helps the heart respond to life's "valleys." The Psalmist states: "I will sing unto the Lord as long as I live." This means always, not just during good times. Singing doesn't have to be in tune, it still uplifts. Even humming brings about good feelings. And have you noticed that you can't whistle and be sad at the same time? There's just something about it that lifts the spirit.

Other tools of joy are laughter and smiles. These are the outward expressions of the joy you feel inside. You cannot say you're joyful and go around with a long face swaddled in gloom and hopelessness. How will others know you are happy?

The ability to laugh uplifts and brings about joy. "Laughter is medicine, preventive against sour thinking, cure for despondency."[3] We are not born with the ability to laugh. It is acquired and developed. It helps us by driving out sadness and pain, and touches the lives of others. Someone once said, "Joy comes, grief goes, we know not how."

People usually would rather be around happy, joyous people who laugh and smile, rather than with those who are constantly sad, joyless and a letdown. Käthe Kollwitz said, "Men without joy seem like corpses." A smile makes others want to smile also. It is very contagious. "Joy and laughter are the gentle rains which keep hopes green and humans from getting dry and sere."[4]

Nehemiah 8:10 states, " . . . the joy of the Lord is your strength." How true! Genuine joy brings us strength to carry out God's work (our mission), and to live for Him. It puts us in the mood for service. We work better and are more productive when we are joyful. Joy also gives us the strength to say no to Satan and his tricks.

Joy gives us the boldness and courage to take a stand for Jesus Christ, and to tell others about His power to save. It gives us the courage to face the storms in this world, and to defy them.

Joy gives us the freedom to enjoy, love and accept others. It also uplifts those around us. Kate Douglas Wiggin puts it this way: "Never miss a joy in this world of trouble—that's my theory! . . . Happiness, like mercy, is twice blest: it blesses those most intimately associated with it and it blesses all those who see it, hear it, feel it, touch it or breathe the same atmosphere."

Joy brings about a change in your life that makes you a better Christian. "Under the joy of the Spirit, a man may act far differently than normal. He can have a song when otherwise he would be sad, be courageous when usually he would be afraid, or show kindness when typically he would react with resentment."[5] This kind of joy cannot be bought or inherited. The Holy Spirit gives it freely to everyone who gives his life to Jesus Christ.

Unfortunately, some Christians lose their joy. Where they were once jubilant, joyous, and full of life, they now walk around with sullen faces, as if the whole world is against them. Their anemic and lukewarm lives do not attest to the presence of the Holy Spirit in them. Somehow through the years, it seems they've lost the first love they once found in Christ. In short, they've become bitter, joyless people determined to make life miserable not only for themselves, but also for others around them.

Several things rob us of joy. The first of these is unconfessed sins. The story of David is a good example. David really understood the burden of unconfessed sins. He first committed adultery, then committed murder to cover up his adultery. The Bible tells us for months he refused to confess these sins, and during this time, the book of Psalms gives us an insight of what went on in his life because of these unconfessed sins. Psalms 32:3–4 talks about how his unconfessed sins impaired his health. His bones waxed old, he roared (whined and complained) all day long, he couldn't sleep (insomnia), had excessive sweating, and was tormented inside. Psalms 51, verses 8 and 12 speak about his bones being broken and his joy taken away.

The good thing about this story is that David did repent. In Psalm 51, verses 8 and 12, David asked the Lord to make him to hear joy and gladness, so that the bones which had been broken could rejoice. He also asked the Lord to restore the joy of his salvation.

When we harbor unconfessed sins, this robs us of the joy we should be enjoying as children of the living God. When we confess our sins, Christ forgives us and the Holy Spirit in us restores the joy we have lost.

Other things that rob us of our joy are neglecting the Word, our personal time with the Lord, and fellowship with other Christians. All of these are essential for our growth as Christians and when we neglect them, this robs us of the joy we should be experiencing in the Spirit.

Right now you may be saying, "How can I sing or be joyful when nothing seems to work in my life? My marriage is breaking up, my kids are disrespectful and in trouble with the police, I've been diagnosed with cancer, and on top of it all, I can't pay my mortgage on time—what is there to be joyful about?" Let me tell you, a personal and genuine relationship with the Lord brings about joy that nothing in this world can destroy. It brings us joy that is life-giving. It gives strength, courage, boldness, and freedom. It takes the place of gloom, sadness and unhappiness in our lives.

Philippians 4:4 admonishes us to rejoice in the Lord always—not only when things are going fine in our lives, but <u>always,</u> even in bad times. The real test of our faith and our trust in Jesus Christ is when people (especially those who don't know Him) see the joy radiating on our faces or through our singing, daily through good and bad times. This fruit of the Spirit must be growing constantly and reproducing in our lives.

Gloom and bitterness will not draw others to Christ Jesus. In fact, it will push people away from you and away from salvation. Remember, part of our service to others includes leading them toward Jesus, not away from Him.

All around you today there are people who are lonely and hurting. They need to know Jesus Christ as their friend and Savior. They need to know about the "unspeakable" joy that only He can give. Why not give them a dose of the Joy of the Lord? Starting today, let them see the joy that nothing can destroy—not loneliness, pain, sickness, or disappointment. Let them see in you the Joy of the Lord!

Prayer: Lord Jesus, forgive me for _____. Today, I pray with David, "Cleanse me from my sins and restore unto me the joy of thy salvation." Help me to come to You daily in Your Word and through daily prayer and thanksgiving. Holy Spirit, may Your joy fill me to overflowing, so that those around me can benefit, and in this way, they may come to know You personally. Amen.

Thoughts: Joy is a net of love by which you can catch souls.
—Mother Teresa

Joy is the most infallible sign of the presence of God.
—Leon Bloy

Notes

1. Leslie Flynn, *The Gift of Joy* (Wheaton, IL: Victor Books, 1980), p. 10.
2. Ibid., p. 30.
3. Rabbi Samuel Silver, *How to Enjoy This Moment* (New York: Cornerstone Library, 1971), p. 51.
4. Ibid., p. 52.
5. Flynn, *The Gifts of Joy,* p. 13.

1 Peter 3:8–9—Finally, be ye all of one mind, having compassion one of another, love as brethren, be pitiful, be courteous, not rendering evil for evil, or railing for railing: but contrawise blessing; knowing that ye are thereunto called, that ye should inherit a blessing.

31
Compassion

One of the most extraordinary examples of compassion I have ever come across was a painting I saw in an antique shop some years ago. It was a picture of a little girl who had done something wrong and had been told to stand in the corner, facing the wall, and her little dog went and stood with her in the corner. What a picture of compassion!

It is the "Christian" thing to empathize with other people in their needs, and to listen patiently to stories of their disappointments, misfortunes and heartbreaks; however, if we do not know what it means to be disappointed, heartbroken, or "in the dumps," our compassion for them is incomplete.

It is difficult to get advice from a person who has never walked in your shoes, and who hasn't a clue about what you are going through. When we ourselves come face to face with personal tragedies, hurts, and disappointments, our best compassion comes forth in time to help others going through their own tragedies, hurts, and disappointments and to offer them hope.

In the movie *The Doctor*, William Hurt plays a doctor at a teaching hospital, who realizes after he himself is diagnosed with cancer, just how it feels to be sick and at the mercy of others, and this reaction brings about major changes in the way he treats his patients afterward. It also changes the way he teaches the interns who would become doctors.

If you've never been confined to a hospital bed and have never had to use a bedpan, or been given an enema, or had an NG tube or catheter inserted, it is difficult for you to understand just how your patients feel or how embarrassing it might be having those procedures done to them.

Webster's Dictionary defines compassion as a sympathetic consciousness of others' distress together with a desire to alleviate it. Someone puts it simply, "Compassion is to suffer with." Our compassion causes us to "suffer" with the person going through a particular distress.

Before my husband left me, I didn't realize what people who were separated from their spouses or divorced had to face, and I had no compassion for "people like that." Then it happened to me! My husband asked for a divorce.

It felt like being hit by a Mack truck! I couldn't believe what was happening to me and I thought surely, nobody understood what I was going through. Except for two friends, my "friends" deserted me like rats leaving a sinking ship, especially those who were Christians. It appeared that even my own family had deserted me.

The day the policeman brought my divorce papers is indelibly embedded in my memory. I felt like a criminal, and wanted to run and hide.

The pain, loneliness and abandonment felt like a thousand swords plunging deep into my heart. Along with these feelings, I also felt humiliated and ashamed because I was the wife of a minister. This kind of thing didn't happen to Christians, let alone the wives of ministers of the Gospel—or so I thought.

I tried every trick in the book to get my husband to come back to me and my son, but nothing seemed to work. In my agony, I turned to food and TV to dull the pain, but it seemed the hurting would never end. In the midst of my pain and humiliation, I cried out to Jesus Christ and He heard me.

One day a friend gave me a passage in the Bible to read. It was Mark 14:32–42. The Bible tells us in this passage that in the Garden of Gethsemane, while Jesus prayed for what He knew was ahead, His disciples slept. As He prayed, He was in such agony, the Bible tells us, that His sweat fell as drops of blood.

There in that garden, He felt the pain, betrayal, loneliness and abandonment. Most importantly, He felt the shame and humiliation. After all, this was the Son of God, and He was going to be crucified, one of the vilest ways an individual could be executed in those days. In addition, He would be crucified in the company of common thieves, by the same people He had come to save.

In the Garden there was no one to comfort Him or to tell Him it was going to be okay, not even His nearest and dearest friends. In fact the Bible tells us that He cried, "My God, my God, why hast thou forsaken me?" In His pain and agony He felt that even God Himself, His Beloved Father, had turned His back on Him! Oh, how lonely He must have felt at that moment.

As I read that story, it suddenly became crystal clear to me— Jesus Christ, the Son of God, went without comfort in that Garden that night, so that I could be comforted. It gave me such a reassuring feeling to know that He understood all those feelings I was going through—after all, He had felt those same feelings and even more, in the Garden of Gethsemane. And because of this, He had compassion for me.

I didn't have to cry or feel sorry for myself anymore. My Lord Jesus Christ had taken on these feelings on my behalf in the Garden that night. I didn't have to allow feelings of betrayal, abandonment, humiliation and shame to weigh me down anymore.

Because of Christ's compassion for me and because I have had the experience of separation and divorce, I am now better equipped to say with assurance to someone suffering these painful feelings, "I know what you are going through. I too have felt that pain, betrayal, loneliness and abandonment, but let me assure you, the hurting will stop. Give them all to Jesus Christ and let Him stand in the gap for you. I know with certainty that He comforts us and heals the scars left by bitter experiences. Allow Him to do that for you today."

You may be passing through very hard times today. Your goal should be learning how to endure, so that God can use you to minister to others who might be undergoing similar problems. Hardships can and do serve a positive purpose.

Have you lost a loved one? You are equipped to reach out with compassion to console the bereaved.

Have you come face to face with personal tragedies and pain? Use them today to reach out to others who might be going through similar tragedies and pains. In other words, put your misfortunes to use! Someone once said, "Adversity causes some men to break; others to break records."

Usually those who have suffered the most and survived are best able to reach out to people who are hurting and to bring them comfort and hope. Our trials and tribulations equip us with special tools like empathy, love and compassion because we've been there and do understand what the other person is going through. 2 Corinthians 1:3–4 states: "Blessed be God, even the Father of our Lord Jesus Christ, the Father of mercies, and the God of all comfort; Who comforteth us in all our tribulation, that we may be able to comfort them which are in any trouble, by the comfort wherewith we ourselves are comforted of God."

This brings me to an important thought: We should thank the Lord for our trials, disappointments and pain because God is preparing us for future ministries to our patients, their families, our coworkers, and others around us. The "preparation" might be very difficult to understand right now, but remember, God has a plan for your life, and He doesn't make mistakes!

Prayer: Dear Lord, thank You for my adversities, because they prepare me for ministry to my patients, their families, and those I come in contact with daily. Please sensitize my heart with Your love and compassion so that I can truly reach out to those who are hurting today, and make a difference in their lives. Thank You again for calling me into the ministry. Amen.

Thought: There is nothing more beautiful than a rainbow, but it takes both rain and sunshine to make a rainbow. If life is to be rounded and many-colored like the rainbow, both joy and sorrow must come of it. Those who have never known anything but prosperity and pleasure become hard and shallow, but those whose prosperity has been mixed with adversity become kind and gracious.

—Author Unknown

Matthew 6:14–15—For if ye forgive men their trespasses, your heavenly Father will also forgive you: But if ye forgive not men their trespasses, neither will your Father forgive your trespasses.

32
Forgiveness

"I will never forgive you for what you did to me!" Have you ever said these words in anger after someone wronged you? We all have at one time or another.

The dictionary defines "to forgive" as "to cease to feel resentment against (an offender); to pardon."

We have all been hurt before and the things that usually hurt us fall into eight categories: annoyances, disappointments, ridicule, humiliation, abandonment, betrayal, deception, and abuse.

Annoyances

Annoyances are occurrences that hurt our feelings. For example, a driver who rudely cuts ahead of you in traffic and then flips you off, or a shopper ahead of you in a long line who has 11 items, and is standing in the "nine items or less" express line. These actions hurt us slightly and can be quickly forgiven or ignored.

Disappointments

Disappointments come in two distinct categories—in circumstances when things don't work out the way we expected;

and in people when they let us down. Examples of disappointments are when the Head Nurse refuses to give you a well-deserved promotion, or when a friend writes you a poor evaluation. The actions might bring pain, but the hurt is temporary and can be easily forgiven and forgotten.

Ridicule

Ridicule involves laughing "at" instead of "with" someone, and usually comes in the form of labels and stereotypes. These actions go deeper than the first two categories, and may leave long and lasting effects on the lives of people.

Humiliation

Humiliation usually goes hand in hand with ridicule. It is any action that hurts your pride and dignity, and makes you look small, especially before your peers. It causes embarrassment, the feeling of degradation, helplessness and hopelessness.

Abandonment

This is when an emotional or physical bond is broken between someone and a significant person in their life, for example, when a "deadbeat" father leaves his wife and children alone to suffer, not caring what happens to them; or when a woman leaves her husband for his best friend. The space left by these cases of abandonment is very difficult to fill, and they leave deep pain and a void that might take a lifetime to heal and forgive.

Betrayal

Nothing is more painful than the betrayal of a friend or someone near and dear to you; it feels like being stabbed in the back by someone you've trusted. A betrayal breaks a vow, a promise, and a trust. An example of betrayal is when someone you've helped, or gone out on a limb for, turns against you. Another example is when a close friend betrays your confidence and tells others what you've told her in secret. This feeling of betrayal is usually caused by someone you trusted, like a close friend, a family member, or even those who claim to be sisters or brothers in Christ. The wounds caused by betrayal run very deep, and therefore usually take a long time to heal and forgive.

Deception

Deception often goes along with betrayal. When you are deceived or lied to by someone you've trusted, it damages your ability to trust others. A good example of deception is when a wife finds out that her husband has lived a double life for years.

Abuse

Abuse comes in many forms. A person can be abused physically, emotionally, or sexually, and this includes domestic abuse, child abuse and neglect, spousal abuse, and pure brutality, like the crimes committed by Hitler on the Jews during the Holocaust. Abuse can be brought upon by a friend, spouse, parent, teacher, religious leader, or by a total stranger. No matter who caused the abuse, it damages self-esteem and self-worth, and leaves you with feelings of guilt, shame and pain that seem to last forever, and these can go on throughout your adult life and may affect future relationships.

The hurt and pain caused by annoyances, disappointments, ridicule and humiliation can be forgiven easily, but others, like abandonment, betrayal, deception and abuse, run deep and are slow and hard to forgive and let go of. These hurtful memories can linger on and on, and ruin the lives of many.

There is no question that to forgive is the good, Christian, honorable and morally right thing to do, yet when it comes down to actually forgiving a <u>real</u> person who has caused you <u>real</u> pain—especially when you didn't deserve that pain, that's another story! As C. S. Lewis aptly put it, "We all agree that forgiveness is a beautiful idea until we have to practice it."

True forgiveness is very difficult. Perhaps the most difficult thing I have had to do was to say "I'm sorry" to someone whom I felt didn't deserve my forgiveness.

It is difficult to forgive. When a person is hurt or betrayed, naturally the first thing that comes to his mind is getting even. That person who hurt him has to pay for the pain he's caused him. An eye for an eye, or in some cases, a head for an eye.

The pain eventually leads to hatred, and hatred distorts the thinking and makes him want evil and terrible things to happen to the other person, even if that person is a family member or former close friend. This is where the thought of revenge comes in.

We think that revenge will bring some satisfaction to the soul, and at the same time put the other person in his place. As you and I know, it doesn't work out that way. Revenge is never sweet or satisfying, and when there is hatred, everybody loses. It damages and destroys lives and relationships.

The more you nurse that grudge, nourish it and play with it, the more the hate festers and spreads. Unfortunately, some people spend their whole lives trying to pay others back for the pain caused them.

"What does it cost to incubate hatred? It will cause a man to lose friends; a merchant to lose customers; a doctor, patients; an attorney, clients. In addition to corroding a disposition, harbored hatred can elevate blood pressure, upset digestive works, ulcerate a stomach, or bring on a nervous breakdown."[1] Like an ulcer, hatred and revenge eat up your insides, and eventually sap up your very life.

Insomnia, muscle spasms, neurotic disorders, coronaries, cancer, and migraine headaches are also considered to be directly connected with incubating, harboring, or nurturing hatred. Hatred is, in a sense, a slow suicide!

"To carry anger against anyone is to poison your own heart, administering more toxin every time you replay in your mind the injury done to you."[2] You cannot hurt others without hurting yourself. Booker T. Washington put it best when he said, "I will let no man drag me down so low as to make me hate him." Yes, hatred and revenge lower a person to the level of the enemy.

It never ceases to amaze me about how quick children are to forgive. One minute they are saying, "I hate you," or "I'll never play with you again," and the next minute they are back together with that person—playing, as if nothing had happened. Why can't adults be like that?

It is indeed very difficult to forgive, but the Bible admonishes us to forgive, and to do so, not only once or twice, but 70 x 7. That's 490 times!

Not only is it very difficult to forgive, it is also very costly. It will cost you a price to forgive someone who has betrayed, deceived, abused, or humiliated you. Forgiving him may cost you a damaged ego, pride and dignity. To forgive him means you have to voluntarily accept the responsibility for the pain he has cost you. This is a tremendous price to pay, but as Christians, we have an obligation to do so.

It was costly for Jesus Christ to forgive us. It cost Him His life on the cross. He is our ultimate role model for forgiveness. God also paid a tremendous price when He allowed His beloved Son to take our place on the cross. Surely, forgiving our enemies is a very small price, compared to the price He had to pay for our own forgiveness.

Yes, forgiveness is difficult and costly, but the Bible tells us we must forgive others—this is a direct command from God.

To forgive means no longer wanting to punish people who have hurt us, knowing that we can never truly pay them back the pain they cause us. It is the inner peace we feel when we stop trying to pay back, and leave everything in God's hands. He tells us in Romans 12:19, "Vengeance is mine, I will repay. . . . " Who is better equipped to repay, you or God? God, of course.

To forgive is to accept the fact that nothing we can do to punish others will help us, heal us or stop the pain they've caused us.

To forgive is letting go of whatsoever we think people have done to us, and moving on with our lives. It involves letting go of the excess emotional baggage we carry around, baggage that holds us back, weighs us down, and keeps us from becoming productive Christians in service for the Lord.

To forgive means letting go of those terrible emotions that are attached to memories of our pasts. I don't believe that a person can have "total amnesia," and completely forget every wrong done to them, but when we truly forgive, we no longer feel intense anger, hatred, resentment, and bitterness toward our enemies for the wrong they've done to us. We now recognize that what happened to us does not have to determine what will take place in our lives in the future. The past is gone forever and can no longer hurt us.

To forgive is to put to better use the energy once consumed by holding grudges, and "holding in" anger, hatred and resentment, and instead using our time and energy to reach out to others who need us. It is realizing that we have better things to do with our lives. Only in this way can we break the vicious cycle of pain and abuse that surrounds unforgiveness.

We've discussed the damage unforgiveness, hatred, and revenge can do to a person. Now let's see what true forgiveness can do for you.

Forgiveness makes you a stronger person. It takes strength and integrity to forgive someone who has deliberately caused you pain. It is easy to hate, but to forgive others takes strength.

Forgiveness is freedom from bondage. When we hold a grudge against another person, in essence we put ourselves in bondage. My pastor, Billy Epperhart, describes it as you with your arms around the other person—his arms are free and he can freely move around and go on about his business, but you can't. You might think you have him in bondage, but in reality, you are the one in bondage. True freedom can only come about when you let go and release that person.

Forgiveness frees us from our past and sets our eyes toward the future, and our ministry to our patients and their families.

Lastly, forgiveness heals the pain from the wounds of our past— wounds we didn't deserve in the first place. Instead of being victims for the rest of our lives, it gives us victory. It brings about reconciliation, and restores relationships; and in this way, stops the bitterness and resentments that ruin fellowship.

The Bible commands us not only to forgive our enemies, but also love them and to be kind to them. "Forgiving them is one thing— but do I have to be kind to them too?" Yes, loving them and being kind to them is also a command. This means holding out your hand to the person who did you wrong, and inviting him to be your friend again. This is a difficult thing for anyone to do, but we must do so if we want to say goodbye to the hatred, bitterness and resentment.

The standard we follow when we forgive is "just as God in Christ also has forgiven us." Only God can give us the insight to see our enemy as a person in need of forgiveness. Only God can make us truly love our enemy.

When God forgives us, He promises to remove our wrongdoings from us "as far as east is from west." He forgets. He doesn't bring it up again two weeks later to open up old wounds. We too must let go of the hurt, and move on with our lives.

In his book *Forgive and Forget*, Lewis B. Smedes tells us that a clear sign that you've forgiven your enemy is when you recall memory of that person who hurt you, and instead of thinking revenge, you feel the power to help him again, and to wish him well! That, my friends, is true forgiveness.

Is there a family member who has hurt you terribly in your past, and whom you have never really forgiven? If so, release that person today and forgive him.

Is there a colleague who has lied to others about you or has said or written terrible things that ruin your reputation? If so, release that person today and allow healing into your life.

Is there a friend who has tried to destroy or abuse you? Let go of the pain right now, so that the hatred, resentment and unforgiveness cannot truly and eventually destroy your life.

Did your spouse deceive you in some way and have you vowed to never forgive that wrong? Forgive him/her today—let go and let God mend that relationship.

Do it today, before it's too late, and before any more damage is done. And let our prayer be today, along with St. Francis of Assisi:

Lord, make me an instrument of Your peace
Where there is hatred, let me sow love;

Where there is injury, pardon;
Where there is discord, unity;
Where there is doubt, faith;
Where there is despair, hope;
Where there is darkness, light;
Where there is sadness, joy.
O Divine Master,
Grant that I may not so much
seek to be consoled, as to console;
To be understood, as to understand;
To be loved, as to love.
For it is in giving, that we receive;
It is in pardoning, that we are pardoned;
And it is in dying, that we are born to
eternal life. Amen.

Prayer: Heavenly Father, forgive me for my unforgiveness. Today, I choose to let go of my painful past and the hurtful memories I have carried around for so long. I lay them at Your feet and leave them there. Fill me with love for others, especially for _____, who has hurt me so much. Help me to forgive him/her today. And Lord, forgive me for all the pain I have caused others. Help them to forgive me. Let me be peacemaker where I live and work. Thank You for Your love that sustains me each day. Amen.

Thought: We are to love, accept and forgive people as individuals, as a person for whom Christ died. That man whom you may find so difficult to forgive, is of infinite worth to God. His Son died for that individual.

—Helen Kooiman

Notes

1. David Augsburger, *The Freedom of Forgiveness, 70 x 7* (Chicago, IL: Moody Press, 1970), p. 14.
2. Patrick D. Miller, *A Little Book of Forgiveness: Challenges and Meditations for Anyone with Something to Forgive* (New York: Viking, 1994), p. 15.

Leviticus 27:30—And all the tithe of the land, whether of the seed of the land, or of the fruit of the tree, is the Lord's: it is holy unto the Lord.

33
Giving

There are many good reasons why we should give. First of all, the Word of God commands us to do so. It is not a question of whether "to give or not to give." To give is not an option. It is a direct command from God. If we want to obey Him, we must give.

These are some of the statements in the Bible about giving: "Give and it shall be given unto you" (Luke 6:38); "Give to him who asketh thee, and from him that would borrow of thee turn not thou away" (Matthew 5:42); "Freely ye have received, freely give" (Matthew 10:8b).

God Himself emphasized the act of giving, by being the ultimate giver. He gave us His Son to take our place on the cross. He has given us a chance to become part of His family. He gives us eternal life. He has given us comfort in crises, peace in the storm, and joy in the face of hardship. He provides shelter, food, and clothing. He has also given us talents and gifts—both natural and spiritual. And He has given these things freely, to people who sometimes don't deserve His benevolence.

Another reason why we should give is because, as the Bible tells us, if we give, we will receive. Luke 6:38 also tells us, "Give, and it shall be given unto you; good measure, pressed down, and shaken together, and running over, shall men give into your bosom. For with the same measure that ye mete withal it shall be measured to you again." If you give selflessly to others, you will also be given your heart's desires.

Giving also blesses. There is something about giving—you cannot do it without feeling very good about yourself. When we give to others the way God expects us to, He in turn gives us our needs, and does so abundantly. He gives us a sort of refund that is more precious and more valuable than the tax refund we get from the government.

Jesus is described in the Book of Acts in this way: "He went about doing good." Jesus gave to us in numerous ways—through His healing, His teachings, and His love for us. As Christian nurses, we too must give to others.

Giving emulates Christ Jesus. He gave His life for us on the cross, and took our shame because He loved us so very much. But that's not all that He gave us. He has given believers like you and me salvation and a chance for eternal life. He also gave us the Holy Spirit, to be our Comforter, Helper and Counselor. He loves us so much!

Our goals for giving to others should be in order to show our love for God, to glorify Him and to show our obedience to His Word. These things make us want to reach out, and to give to those in need.

People have different motives for giving to others. Some of these motives are wrong and others are right. People give for their own glory and greed. A good example of this is in the story about Ananias and Sapphira, who pretended to be generous people by selling their property, and giving the money to the apostles; but as the story goes, they withheld part of the money they had donated, and this led to their demise. Some people give because they want to impress their peers. Ananias and Sapphira did just that. As Christians, we sometimes give in order to impress the people around us, rather than to bring glory to God.

Others give only because come tax time, they will get a large tax deduction. It is okay to get what's coming to you, but if your only motive for giving is for tax deduction, to impress others, or for your own glory and greed, this is wrong. When we have wrong motives, we become selfish, proud and greedy, and this does not please or glorify God.

Our motives in giving should be because we want to please God and so that He can use us as His instruments to bless others. We must give not merely out of duty, but because God wants us to. Other good motives are: to lay up treasures in heaven (Matthew 6:19–21), and to reach the world for Jesus Christ.

Matthew 10:8b admonishes us to give freely or voluntarily. No one can force or coerce us to give. Giving has to be a voluntary act done in obedience to God's will. Proverbs 11:24 tells us that when we give freely, we will receive. The Bible also tells us that when we give, we should do so generously (Romans 12:8), and in secret (Matthew 6:4). We should not boast, or draw attention to our giving; neither should we keep a record. Lastly, when we give, we should do so cheerfully without grumbling or complaining, because God loves a cheerful giver (2 Corinthians 9:7).

Everything we own belongs to God (Colossians 1:16–17). He owns our money and personal belongings, our gifts and talents, our minds, bodies and even the time we have to spend. Everything we have, He owns. What He has done is to entrust these things to our care. In other words, we are merely stewards.

A steward is a manager or overseer of another person's property. We have been placed (by God), as managers and overseers over His property. We are responsible for taking care of these properties. He expects us to be faithful and wise stewards and to properly manage what He has entrusted to our care. One of these days, we will have to give an account of what we did with the things God has so graciously placed in our care, while here on earth (Romans 14:12).

When we tithe, we offer a part of the substances God has given to us, back to Him. When we tithe, we are in essence saying to God that we acknowledge the fact that everything we own is His.

The word "tithe" comes from an Old English term which means "a tenth." God expects us to give a tenth of the first fruits of our labor to Him (Proverbs 3:9–10). He reminds us of the reward we will receive for obeying Him with our tithes—He promises to provide for our needs in an abundant manner that will astonish us and others. He doesn't necessarily say we will be wealthy or millionaires, but He promises to take care of our needs. He says He will fill our barns and vats. This is a promise.

In Malachi 3:10–12, God makes a deal with us. He tells us that if we give Him our tithes and offerings, there are some things that will take place in our lives. He promises us to pour out a blessing so vast, that there shall not be room enough to receive it. He also promises to rebuke the devourer (Satan) for our sakes, so that he will not destroy the fruits of our ground. Neither will our vine cast her fruit before its time. And that's not all! He also promises that everyone will call us blessed.

He promises to do all these things if we give him back what already belongs to Him. He is telling us today to test Him and see if He doesn't do all He has promised us and even more. So many of us lose out on the special blessings we should be receiving from God, because we refuse to take Him at His word.

We should offer God the tithe of our money, and we must do it voluntarily and cheerfully. This can be done by giving a tenth of our money (in addition to extra for offerings) to our local churches, para-church groups, missionaries, and those around us who are in need.

We should also tithe our time. A tenth of 24 hours a day is only two hours and forty minutes. Some of us spend more than that amount of time in front of our TVs, playing golf, or gossiping. We must dedicate this time to work of the Lord. Things to do include: attending church or Bible study, spending personal time with the Lord, meeting specific needs of our patients and their families, sharing our faith with others, helping the needy, and encouraging others.

We should also offer God our gifts and talents to be used for His service. Every Christian has at least one gift or talent that can be used to serve others.

It is okay to give our possessions, money, time, talents, and gifts in service for Jesus Christ, but these things are not sufficient. As Paul tells us in Romans 12:1, we must also present our bodies as a living sacrifice, holy and acceptable, unto God. This is our reasonable service! The best gift we can give to God is the giving of ourselves for His purpose and in His service.

How can you give your body? You can do so by giving your life to Jesus Christ (if you haven't done so already). You can do so by becoming born again (see chapter 41).

You can give Him your eyes—eyes that are sensitive to the needs of your patients and their families. Proverbs 6:16–17 tells us that God hates a proud look. We should strive to get rid of those things that distort our spiritual "vision," such as pride, hatred, prejudices, fears, and our own petty problems. Allow Jesus Christ to give you a perfect 20/20 "vision."

You can give him control of your tongue. One of the marks of a genuine Christian is a tongue that has been brought under the control of the Holy Spirit. When we give the Holy Spirit control over our tongue, He makes us to use it as a tool that encourages, uplifts, builds up and leads others to Jesus.

You can give Him your hands and feet, to use in His service. Hands that will be used in honest work to reach those in need, and feet that will go a distance to reach people for Christ.

You can give Him your heart. Proverbs 4:23 states, "Keep thy heart with all diligence; for out of it are the issues of life." The heart is the focal point of our emotions. It is in the heart that we love and hate, believe or doubt, forgive or seek revenge. Unless the heart is placed under God's control, there will always be trouble. Our heart will either be God's domain, or the devil's playground. Today Jesus Christ is saying, "My Son, give me thine heart" (Proverbs 23:26).

You can also give Him your mind. Paul tells us in Romans 8:6 that the carnal mind is death, and is hostile to God, but the spiritually minded is life and peace. Only God can make our minds spiritual. Isaiah 26:3 tells us that He will keep in perfect peace, those whose minds belong to Him. Do you want life and peace? Give your mind to Him.

Give your whole life to Him along with a portion of your money, gifts, talents and time. He deserves more than our leftovers. He deserves the very best. Today, say along with the songwriters (Frances R. Havergal and Henri A César Malan):

> Take my life and let it be,
> Consecrated, Lord, to Thee;
> Take my hands and let them move,
> At the impulse of Thy love;
> Take my feet and let them be
> Swift and beautiful for Thee;
> Take my voice and let me sing,
> Always, only, for my King;

Take my lips and let them be,
Filled with messages for Thee;
Take my silver and my gold,
Not a mite would I withhold;
Take my love, my God, I pour,
At Thy feet its treasure store;
Take myself, and I will be,
Ever, only, all for Thee.

<u>Prayer:</u> **Father, help me to voluntarily and cheerfully give back to You those things that are rightfully Yours. Make me a faithful steward of all the wonderful gifts, talents, money, possessions and time You have entrusted to my care. May I use these things to bring others to You. One of these days when I stand before You to give an account of what I did with these things, may I hear You say, "You did very well, my good and faithful servant." Thank You again for calling me into your ministry. In Your precious Name, Amen.**

<u>Thought:</u>
> Some think that they have everything
> When riches come their way,
> But that they're poor will be revealed
> On God's accounting day.
> —Henry G. Bosch

2 Chronicles 7:14—If my people, which are called by my name, shall humble themselves, and pray, and seek my face, and turn from their wicked ways; then will I hear from heaven, and will forgive their sin, and will heal their land.

34
Prayer

Some people will only pray when they are in church, in pain or agony, in an accident, when a loved one is sick, when things are not working out for them, or when they want something badly. They seem to use prayer as a form of an SOS signal sent to God, to let Him know that they need Him right away. Even those who aren't Christians, or who do not go to church, will cry out "Help me, God," when things aren't working out for them. It is okay to cry out to God for help, but prayer is more than crying out to God, praying in church, or saying grace before meals.

The word "prayer" derives from the Latin verb *precari*, which means "to ask." Prayer is a dialogue (a two-way conversation) between you and God where you speak and listen to God, and He listens and speaks to you. It is your "quality" time together.

We pray because we realize our own inadequacies, and recognize the need to depend on One who is greater and wiser than we are, and who has a power greater than our own.

When we come to God in prayer, our needs are met by His divine arrangement. Our circumstances are exposed as we await His intervention with anticipation. Our lives are also exposed, and He forgives us our sins.

Prayer is our source of spiritual guidance, growth and power, directly from God. It is a time when we have communication with Him, allowing Him to enrich our lives. It is also a time of fellowship when we enjoy our special time with Him.

Prayer is a personal contact with God. He is not out there in space, He is with us constantly. All we have to do to catch His attention is to reach out to Him. Like the lady in the Bible who reached out and touched Jesus Christ, we too can reach out and touch Him. Even in these noisy, busy, and fast-moving times, He still feels our touch when we reach out to Him in prayer. We are very important to Him, and He cares for us. He knows our needs, wants and even our desires, and when we come into His presence, our prayers tap into His bountiful resources.

Who needs to pray? You, I, and everyone. Now more than ever, we need to pray. As Christian nurses, we need to pray for not only ourselves, but also for our families, homes and those we come in contact with daily—our coworkers, our patients and their families.

We ought to pray during bad times and good times—when things are sunny or bleak. We ought to pray when our patients are sick, and when they recover. We ought to pray when an ambulance goes past us on the highway or when the operator calls out "Code Zero" or "Code Blue" on a patient. We ought to pray continuously. First Thessalonians 5:17 teaches us to pray without ceasing—this means in both good and bad times. Your whole life must be permeated by prayer. Prayer is not a luxury, it is a necessity for everyone who calls himself a Christian! One of the most important components of prayer is faith. Mark 11:24 states, "Therefore I say unto you, what things soever ye desire, when you pray, believe that ye receive them, and ye shall have them." Faith is praying with anticipation. We must expect something to happen when we pray, or else what's the use of praying? When we pray, we must believe that God is real and all-knowing, and that He is aware of our needs. We must believe that He hears us when we pray, and that He answers prayers, or else our prayers are a waste of time.

We say we have faith when we pray, yet when that prayer is answered immediately we act very surprised! Why do we do that? Is it because we really didn't believe that God could grant our requests, or is it because we don't believe He can still perform miracles in the lives of people today? No matter what your answer is, this is the fact: God is real and He hears us when we pray, therefore when we go to Him in prayer we must do so with the belief that He will answer those prayers.

Does God really answer prayers? The answer is a big YES! He answers prayers in several ways: "yes," "no," "wait," and "I have something better for you."

God may say "Yes, I will give you what you asked for." That "yes" might come immediately, or it might come a year from the time you asked. Either way, He knows what is best for you and His timing is incredible.

God may say, "No, I cannot give you what you asked for." There might be several reasons why His answer is no. Perhaps you asked in the wrong way. 2 Chronicles 7:14 teaches that we must humble ourselves, pray and seek God's face, and turn away from our wicked ways, then He will hear us from heaven, forgive our sins and heal our land. Perhaps you were not humble, or the time is wrong. Perhaps there are unforgivenesses or unconfessed sins in your life. No matter what the reasons are, be reminded—God is in control. He sees the future, and therefore knows what is good or bad for us! His decisions are by far more reliable than ours.

Another way God answers us is, "Not now, wait until later." Again, His timing is best. He might tell us to wait for several reasons. One of these reasons could be that He wants to prepare us for the coming blessing. Maybe we need to grow and mature as Christians, before He can trust us with that precious blessing, or maybe we need to learn a lesson in patience. Our duty is to wait on Him and to continue to pray as we await His answer.

God may also say to us, "I have something better for you!" Sometimes He substitutes what we asked for with something that is better by far. At other times, he might decrease our need for that particular thing, or put us in a position to not have a need for it.

Yes, friends, God does answer prayers. Sometimes we think He doesn't answer, because we take our own plans and agenda to Him and expect Him to put His seal of approval on them and when this doesn't work, we say He didn't answer!

When it seems like He doesn't hear you, don't stop praying. Remember that God is still in control and His timing is precise and accurate. Also examine yourself—have you confessed all your sins? What is the motive for your petition? Do you want that particular thing because it will make you richer or more famous? Is it something you want, or something you really need? As you answer these questions, keep in mind that our selfishness, unforgiveness, and other sins can be hindrances in our communication with our Father, and that God will not say "yes" if it is not in His own plan or purpose for our lives, or if it doesn't bring glory to His name.

It is important to mention here the significance of our private time with the Lord. It is good to pray in church, at meals, or have a time of family prayer and worship, but it is of vital importance to set aside a time to be with our Lord. You must choose a time when you can be alone and undisturbed, to pray. Some people like to pray late at night, just before bedtime. I like early in the morning because for me, it is quiet and calm and I can be undisturbed for about an hour.

Psalms 17:15 states that our first thoughts (when we wake up from sleep) should be about God. This is a great head start, because our first thoughts and attitudes usually set the mood for the rest of the day. If you wake up with a terrible disposition, chances are it will be carried over through the rest of the day at home or at work. When you start the day with the Lord in prayer, you are starting the day on the right foot. It is good to greet each morning with a personal relationship with the Lord, and being in His presence. This will prepare us to meet the world, with its stresses, frustrations, hardships, temptations, and other problems we will be facing that day. A Christian nurse, working with patients in life and death situations, needs to start the day with the Lord.

For years, I neglected my personal time with the Lord and it took its toll on my life, my family and in my work. About four years ago I started a daily prayer time, and it has made an incredible difference in my spiritual life and my relationship with my family and the people I come in contact with daily. This time has been rewarding and wonderful. I urge you to start a daily prayer time if you aren't already doing so. You will be amazed what a difference it will make in your life.

Below is the model I use for my personal prayer time. I hope it will help you to start your own model for your prayer time.

My prayer time usually lasts 30 minutes to an hour a day. I turn off the TV and unplug the telephone in my room. My son knows that this is my time with the Lord, and he tries to not disturb me.

I start by reading passages from the Bible. My objective is to complete the Bible, so I read two or three chapters from the Old and New Testaments daily, and take notes. After the Bible reading, which usually lasts about 15 to 20 minutes, I spend about five minutes preparing for my time of prayer. This preparation includes either singing or listening to spiritual music. Then I am ready to pray. There are six items included on my prayer list:

1. Confession of sins
2. Praise and adoration
3. Thanksgiving
4. Intercession for others
5. Petitions of my own
6. A time of silence, meditation

Confessions of sins

I believe that it is significant to confess sins first of all, because I strongly believe that sin will hinder our prayers from reaching God. Proverbs 15:8 and 29 state that God hears the prayer of the righteous and it pleases Him.

God hates sin. It separates us from God, so in order to be in a one to one relationship with Him we must come daily to His presence, confessing our sins and begging for forgiveness; then we can stand boldly in His presence and give Him our petitions.

You must be honest and specific as you examine yourself. Confess sins you know you've committed by words, thoughts and deeds—even sins you don't realize you've committed. The Bible tells us if we confess our sins, God is faithful and just to forgive us our sins and cleanse us from all unrighteousness. Confess your sins and beg God's forgiveness, and ask Him for strength to not repeat the sin. We must also accept God's forgiveness. Now you are ready to go to the next step.

Praise and Adoration

God desires to be loved, honored, adored and appreciated by those He has created. In fact, He created us for His glory. He deserves our best praise and adoration.

My son, Jeff, really knows when and how to praise me. Whenever he wants me to do something for him, he says how much he loves me and what a great Mom I am (in fact the best in the world), and I tell you, it works every time!

I am not telling you to give God vain praises when you want something from Him, but He deserves our praises daily. We must lift Him high and put Him where He belongs—above all else. We must tell Him daily just how much we love and appreciate Him. We must say with the Psalmist, "I will bless the Lord at all times: His praise shall continually be in my mouth. My soul shall make her boast in the Lord: the humble shall hear thereof, and be glad. O magnify the Lord with me."

Thanksgiving

Just as He desires praise and adoration, God also desires gratitude for His blessings toward us. We should thank Him for answered prayers, and for the many blessings He has enriched us with. We ought to thank Him for the basic necessities of life, such as shelter, food and clothing. We ought to thank Him for our health. Even if you have minor illnesses, you can still go to work and support your family. If your illness is major, thank Him that you are still alive, and if you are on your death bed—still give Him thanks because He has a place in heaven, just waiting for you.

There are many other things we can thank Him for: personal possessions like cars, home, money in the bank; family and friends; our job or business; our pastor and church family; our country and its leaders (even if we don't agree with their politics). There are many things to thank God for. It doesn't hurt to make a list.

Counting your blessings daily makes you realize just how much God loves and cares for you. Our prayers of gratitude reach up to Him and opens doors for more blessings into our lives.

Intercession for Others

This involves praying or pleading on behalf of others. The Bible teaches us to bear other people's burdens (Galatians 6:2). When they are sad or in pain, as Christians we should have empathy and compassion for them. When they are happy, we should share in their joy. Praying for them should cover all these areas. We must also be concerned about their spiritual condition. Intercession involves praying for their salvation. Intercessory prayers take your own needs and wants out of the picture (for a while) and make the needs of others a priority.

People we need to intercede for include: our families, friends, coworkers, patients and their families, our church family, and even strangers we encounter or hear about. At times the Holy Spirit will bring to mind the name of a person. You might not understand why, but pray for that person anyway.

James 5:16 tells us, "The effectual fervent prayer of a righteous man availeth much." We need "prayer warriors" who are willing to intercede on behalf of those who are not able to, or do not want to pray for themselves. God can use us to lead these people to Him.

Petition for Yourself

After interceding for others, this is a good time to bring your own petitions before the Lord. Keep your priorities straight. Remember, it is okay to ask Him for anything—big favors and little favors, impossibilities and even easy or simple things like finding a good parking space, for a good day at work, or finding a lost item. Don't only ask for earthly things that are usually temporary, also ask Him for heavenly things which are eternal. Ask for His guidance in making sound and moral decisions. It is okay to cry out to the Lord sometimes—like a kid who cries out to his dad. After all God (our Heavenly Father) cares for us. He cares for our every need.

There is nothing that you cannot take to the Lord. Sometimes we don't pray when we should because we think we are self-sufficient. I remember years ago in Africa, we prayed for almost everything. We prayed for the rains to come so that the crops would grow well that season, or for enough money to buy food and other necessities of life. Then we came to America and instead of praying for things we needed daily, we went to the ATM machine and got money. It seemed like we no longer needed to depend on God for our provisions. That really must have hurt our Heavenly Father!

John 15:7 teaches us that if we abide in Him and His Word abides in us, if we ask anything in the name of Jesus Christ, we will be granted our petition. With this in mind, let us go into God's presence, knowing our prayers will be answered.

A Time of Silence/Meditation

After you give your petition to God, it helps to spend a period of time in silence, in order to listen to what God has to say to you. Use this time for meditation. It doesn't have to be a long time, just a moment when you allow your mind to be occupied with God, and Him alone. It might take a while, but you will begin to see the difference this time will make in your prayer time.

In addition to my personal time with the Lord, another way I have used prayer in my work is praying together with other nurses. In Matthew 18:19-20, Jesus states, "Again, I say unto you, That if two of you shall agree on earth as touching anything that they shall ask, it shall be done for them of my Father which is in heaven. For where two or three are gathered together in my name, there am I in the midst of them."

It is good to pray with other nurses and other people who

love the Lord. Even when it's busy, you can make time to go in a room or even in the nurses' lounge and pray for your patients and their families, your colleagues and for guidance for the rest of the shift. Short, meaningful prayers will avail much not only for ourselves, but also for those placed in our care. Having other nurses as prayer partners is great, because you can intercede for each other, and support each other spiritually. I have been blessed immensely by my prayer partners (Laura Berry, Ruth Kneebone, and Pam Fountain), who have been a source of support and encouragement for me, especially for the years I have been writing this book. I praise the Lord for them. What a difference they have made in my life!

Friends, we need to go daily to the Lord in prayer for our own needs and the needs of others. In prayer, we come face to face with God and our prayers are answered. If you aren't already doing so, I urge you to start today, and see what a difference prayer will make in your life.

Prayer: My Heavenly Father, thank You for making it possible for us to come to You with problems and our petitions knowing that You hear us and answer us. Forgive me today for all the sins I've committed in words, thoughts and deeds. Give me the strength to say no to those sins the next time I encounter them. I praise You because of who You are. Thank You for all the things You've blessed me with. You have been good to me. I pray for my family, my friends, and the patients You have placed in my care. Please meet their needs in Your special way. And Father, please teach me to pray. In the precious Name of Your Son Jesus Christ. Amen.

Thought: The Christian on his knees sees more than the philosopher on tiptoe.

—D. L. Moody

Psalm 91:11—For he shall give his angels charge over thee, to keep thee in all thy ways.

35
Protection

Any nurse who has worked the "graveyard" shift knows how it feels to walk the dark corridors and poorly lit parking lots to get to your car, especially in areas that are not safe. And any nurse who has had to care for patients with highly contagious illnesses, like TB, AIDS, and hepatitis, knows the feeling of uneasiness for fear of cross-contaminations. As we go about our duties, we are mindful of the many things we need protection from. This chapter deals with the way God uses angels to protect us.

Lately there seems to be a craze and a fascination with angels. Everywhere you look there are signs of angels—books, magazines, TV news reports, talk shows, figures of angels, music and collectibles, all relating to angels.

All of a sudden, everyone is talking about seeing and experiencing angels.

The Bible tells us that God has many angels at His command. Angels are mentioned about three hundred times in the Bible, and each time the angels were there to assist people in their spiritual, emotional, and physical struggles.

Webster's Dictionary defines an angel as a spiritual being superior to man in power and intelligence. Angels are not to be confused with the Holy Spirit. The Holy Spirit is the third person of the trinity, and is therefore God. He comes to dwell in us when we become born-again Christians. He is all-knowing, all-powerful, and all-present—all attributes of the Godhead.

An angel is not a god. He appears to people, but does not dwell in people. The Holy Spirit convicts men of sin, teaches us how to live, and strengthens, energizes and empowers us for effective service to others; while the angel is a messenger of God, who comes to serve as a ministering spirit (Hebrews 1:14).

Angels also differ from man. The Bible states that God made man a "little lower than the angels." Man has dominion over the creatures of the earth, but is lower than angels, who are more powerful and have more knowledge than man. Angels are sexless, and do not marry (Matthew 22:30) or procreate. They also do not die.

Good Angels vs. Bad Angels

The book of Revelation tells us about the continuous and bitter conflict between the holy angels that are faithful to God, and the angels of darkness, who are followers of Lucifer.

In the beginning, God created the angels (including Lucifer) for the purpose of glorifying Him, but the Bible tells us that Lucifer wanted to be higher than God. He wasn't satisfied with being God's subordinate. He wanted to dethrone God Himself. Lucifer's pride and conceit caused him to rebel against God and it has been estimated that about a third of the angels may have joined him in this rebellion (Revelation 12:7–9). To this day, Satan and his angels of darkness (or demons, as they are sometimes referred to) are constantly in battle in heaven and here on earth.

Certainly, demonstrations of Satan and his demons are evident on earth today. All you have to do is look around you. There are kids killing other kids; there are troubled areas in all corners of the earth; and there are wars and the rumors of war, and the more world leaders meet to bring peace, the worse things get. There are more divorces, abortions, euthanasia, domestic violence, incest, rape and murders than ever before. There is also an increase in the worship of Satan and a rapid trend towards the New Age movement. There is a spiritual warfare.

There is no question about it—Satan and his angels of darkness are alive and hard at work on earth today. Satan realizes his time is about up and therefore he and his followers are working overtime, to get as many followers as possible to join them into the "everlasting fire" that has been prepared for them (Matthew 25:41).

I seriously believe that because Satan knows his end is near, he and his angels are roaming this earth constantly, and therefore, more and more people are having encounters with holy angels sent by God to minister to them.

Angels Minister

Angels minister to people. They can be visible (be seen physically) or invisible (without us being aware of their presence). Either way, they minister to us. In times of hardships, discouragement, sickness and oppression, angels (God's heavenly messengers) have brought encouragement, hope, peace and deliverance to many people, and have sustained and lifted the spirits of others. "Angels have ministered the message, 'All is well,' to satisfy fully the physical, material, emotional and spiritual needs of the people."[1]

Angels Protect and Deliver

God also uses angels to warn us that we will be held in judgment. Angels came to earth to warn Abraham about what would happen to Sodom and Gomorrah, because of their wickedness. Today, angels still come to warn people of impending danger. God also uses angels to execute His judgment, like the angel who destroyed the Assyrian army (2 Kings, chapter 19), and the one who almost destroyed Jerusalem (1 Chronicles, chapter 21).

Angels Bring Good News

We all know about the angels who appeared to both Mary (the mother of Jesus) and her cousin Elizabeth, bringing the good news of the birth of their sons; and the angels that appeared to the shepherds proclaiming the birth of Jesus Christ, also the one that appeared to Joseph. Today, angels still come bearing the good news of salvation in Christ Jesus.

Worship the Creator, Not the Creature

God sends angels to minister, protect and deliver us, to warn us and to bring us good news, but let us remember that angels (like man) were created by God, and should therefore not be worshiped. Romans 1:24–25 warns us against worshiping the creature rather than the Creator. Only God is worthy of that privilege. "We do not pray to angels. Nor are we to engage in a 'voluntary humility and worshiping' of them. Only the triune God is the object of our worship and of our prayers."[2]

Considering the fascination individuals have with angels today, many people who have refused to accept Jesus Christ as their Lord and Savior are more than willing to embrace angels for protection and deliverance. Remember, angels are messengers sent by the Almighty God. We must place our trust in Him and Him alone, for our protection.

It is not enough that we hang angels around our necks, in our homes, or carry them around with us. We must have the Creator of the angels in our hearts and in our lives. We must first have a personal relationship with the One who sends the angels to protect and deliver us.

God has promised to protect us from danger (both physical and emotional) and also from attacks from Satan and his angels. Satan and his followers are busy out there, but praise God, we have His angels taking charge over us, our loved ones, and our personal belongings.

I have never seen an angel physically, but I have felt the presence of a being looking over my shoulders—looking out for me, warning me and protecting me. I strongly believe that each of us has a guardian angel, sent by God to guide, protect and minister to us.

If you are a believer, expect the presence of the holy angels as you go about your daily duties in service for others. With God we have genuine security and safety from danger, and from the evils of this world.

Prayer: Heavenly Father, thank You for angels You have sent to minister to me. Thank You for Your continuous protection for me, my family and friends, my patients and colleagues, and my personal belongings. The next time I face danger in any form, please remind me that Your angels are around me, looking out for my safety. Thank You for caring for all my needs, even my need for security. Amen.

Thought: Angels are the dispensers and administrators of the divine beneficence toward us. They regard our safety, undertake our defense, direct our ways, and exercise a constant solicitude that no evil befall us.
—John Calvin

Notes

1. Billy Graham, *Angels: God's Secret Agents* (Garden City, NY: Doubleday, 1975), p. 85.
2. Ibid., p. 29.

Genesis 1:27—So God created man in his own image, in the image of God created he him; male and female created he them.

36
Healthy Self-Esteem

Self-esteem is a topic everyone is talking about these days, but what exactly is self-esteem? According to Janet Ohlemacher (*Desperate to Be Needed*), "Self-esteem, used interchangeably with self-worth, self image, and self-acceptance, describes the way we think and feel about ourselves." We all have self-esteem, whether good or bad, high or low, healthy or unhealthy—we all have some form of self-esteem.

There are three basic emotional needs: the need for a sense of belonging, a sense of worth, and a sense of competence. These three areas make up the substance or foundation of the way we think and feel about ourselves. Our appearance, how we perform, and how important we are to significant people in our lives are areas we evaluate ourselves by.

Our Appearance

Our physical appearance has a lot to do with the way we think and feel about ourselves. "How do I look?" is a question we often ask. How other people (especially our peers) react to our appearance is very important to us. This is illustrated by the millions of dollars we spend each year to buy clothes, accessories, makeup and jewelry, and the millions spent each year fixing the nose and ears, and on facelifts, weight loss programs, tummy-tucks, breast augmentation, hair transplants, and other types of self-improvements, in order to be "perfect."

Few of us are happy with the way we look. We feel we are either too fat or too skinny, too tall or too short, too small in some areas of our body, or too big in others.

This feeling of wanting to be "perfect" begins at a very early age. From the moment we are able to sit up by ourselves and to read, we are beset by pictures of "perfect" people on TV, and in books and magazines. We are made to feel that something is wrong with us if we don't look like those "perfect" people. Even the toys we play with send us messages that if we don't look like Barbie or Ken, we are nothing. If we want to be "somebody" or to belong, we have to be "perfect."

How we feel about ourselves changes depending on whether we receive compliments about our appearance, or if we are criticized for the way we look. These feelings come about because we want to belong. If we look different because of our physical appearance, we are not accepted by our peers. We think in order to belong, we must live up to the standards of their "perfect" image.

Our Performance

What we think and feel about ourselves depends on how we perform in comparison with others, especially our peers. "How am I doing?" is a question that is embedded in us from the very beginning. From the day we are born, the comparisons start. They want to know what our Apgar score is, how long we are, and how big we are, compared to the other babies in the nursery.

At home, we are given chores and special responsibilities, and we are rated on how we do these chores and responsibilities. From kindergarten throughout the span of our education, we are rated by our performances. Grades, report cards, awards, promotions, honors lists, and I.Q. tests, all attest to this fact. In our careers, we are also rated on how we perform our duties as nurses, mothers, wives, and Christians, not only by the compliments we receive, but also by the peer evaluations and criticisms of our competence. From these ratings, we formulate our self-image based on our successes and our failures.

Comparison is a form of competitive game. It involves trying to "keep up with the Joneses." We want to be better than others, richer, more attractive, more gifted, more talented, or in a higher social class or position. We allow our self-esteem to either rise or fall, according to where we think we are in comparison to our peers. The thing about this kind of thinking is that there will always be someone who is richer, more beautiful, more talented, or in a higher position or social class than we are. When we compare ourselves with others, it leaves us with either good or bad feelings about ourselves.

Our Importance

How important we are to our parents, family, friends, peers and colleagues influences the way we think and feel about ourselves. The respect, acceptance, admiration and value we receive from these significant people in our lives plays a very important role in how important we think we are.

From birth, the experience of receiving love from our parents forms the building blocks on which we will look at ourselves and see a person of value and worth. If our parents show us that they accept us as we are (warts and all), we begin to see value and worth in ourselves. Good parents teach us to love ourselves just the way we are, even if we are not as "perfect" as the world wants us to be. When we are loved and accepted by our parents, chances are we will be able to love others the way we should.

It is a pity that too many children don't have the luxury of having parents who truly love them, care for them, and accept them the way they are. Without that love and acceptance, an individual craves for these from other people and in the wrong places. Without that sense of value, love and acceptance, a person can be doomed to live with low self-esteem.

As we grow older, we continue to receive messages from our friends, classmates, teachers, and others in the society, about how valuable we are. If we are told that our inadequacies or handicaps in certain areas make us outcasts and unfit, we begin to believe that it is true, and we behave like failures. If we are told by their words and actions, that even with our imperfections, we are "somebody," that too will influence our self-worth.

The messages we receive from outside influence how we feel inside.

As Christians, it is important to note what part God plays in the way we should think about ourselves. When we accept Jesus Christ as our Lord and Savior, we receive a new identity. Second Corinthians 5:17 states, "Therefore if any man be in Christ, he is a new creature: old things are passed away; behold, all things are become new."

When we become born again, we become sons of God, with the same inheritance His Son has. The Bible tells us that we become joint-heirs with Jesus Christ (Romans 8:17). We are now a part of God's family. That makes us "somebody." Our relationship with God (our Heavenly Father) gives us a new sense of belonging.

God loves us very much. He expressed that love for us when He sent His Son to die in our place. His love is unconditional, and He loves us in spite of our shortcomings, inadequacies, and our "imperfect" nature. Even when we let Him down by our words, thoughts and actions, He still loves—enough to sacrifice Jesus for us. That, my friends, is real love! That love validates our sense of belonging.

Our relationship with Jesus Christ makes us worthy. His death on the cross proves that worth. He didn't waste His precious blood on that cross for nothing. He went to the cross voluntarily, because He knew how much we mattered to Him. We are very special to Him. Someone once put it this way: "God doesn't love us because we are valuable, we are valuable because He loves us." His love qualifies us and makes us priceless. In Him alone, we are complete.

We also have a sense of competence because of our relationship with the Holy Spirit. He is our Comforter, Helper and Friend, and our very source of strength. Through Him, we are able to be anything we want to be in the Lord. He empowers us to become the type of Christians God can use in His service. He does this by making us fruitful Christians expressing love, joy, peace, patience, kindness, goodness, faithfulness, gentleness and self-control. He guides us, helps us in our weakness, and intercedes for us. Through Him, we become competent.

Our relationship with God the Father, God the Son, and God the Holy Spirit validates us in all three areas of our basic emotional needs. We belong, have worth, and are competent, because God loves us. No matter how we feel about ourselves, or how others feel about us, to God, our value does not diminish. He values us just the same. Remember that the next time you think you are a "nobody."

Do you want to reclaim your self-esteem, or boost up the way you value yourself? Below are some suggestions.

Accept Yourself As You Are

This is the first step in reclaiming your self-esteem. You are made in the image of God Himself; that makes you very important. You are an original. When God made you, He broke the mold—there is no one else exactly like you, never was, and never will be. This uniqueness makes you very special to God. God loves you just as you are, but He doesn't want you to stay that way forever. He wants you to grow and become all you can be in Him, but you have to take the first step. This involves loving and accepting yourself "as is." Black or white, fat or thin, tall or short, perfect or imperfect—He still loves you and always will. You must also love and accept yourself.

Accepting yourself as you are doesn't mean you shouldn't make self-improvements. Make some changes if that will make you feel better about yourself. There are things about us that we cannot change, such as our race, family and age; but we can improve our appearance, and change our weight, attitudes and habits. Dress better, lose some weight, stop smoking, or go back to school to further your education if that will make you feel better about yourself; but remember even if you do not succeed at these things, God still loves you. You are still valuable to Him.

You are fearfully and wonderfully made (Psalm 139:14). Accept yourself as you are, and love yourself. Be thankful to God for the way you are. Then you can say along with the old Negro saint:

> Maybe I ain't what I want to be,
> But Praise God,
> I ain't what I used to be;
> And I ain't what I'm gonna be.

Don't Compare Yourself with Others

God has blessed you with a lot of potential. He has given you gifts and talents to use in His service—use them, and stop comparing them with others'. He has given each of us different kinds of gifts and talents. Some people have more, others fewer, but we all have something to offer in service to others. Be content with what you have, and develop and use them for God's glory. When we keep our eyes on the other person's gifts and talents and we start to envy them, we take our eyes off God. Envy is a total waste of time and energy that should be spent serving God. Epictetus stated, "He is a wise man who does not grieve for the thing which he has not, but rejoices for those which he has."

Start today with what you have (yourself, "as is"), and grow wherever God has planted you. Remember that there will always be someone else who is more attractive, richer, cleverer, or more talented than you are. Use what God has blessed you with, to bring glory to His name.

Count Your Blessings

If possible make a list of your natural and spiritual gifts and talents. Next, make a list of all the great things God has given you, such as your family, job, friends, house, car, and other blessings. Finally, make a list of all your accomplishments, such as the type of education you have acquired, special job skills, awards you have won, people you have led to Christ, and great strides you've made in your career. Let these things be a constant reminder to you that you are worth something. You are valuable.

Don't Allow Failure to Discourage You

The fear of failure will only keep you from moving forward to better things in your life. Remember, no one is perfect. We all make mistakes. We all have faults and imperfections. Other people's faults may not be visible to the naked eye, but we all have faults. The thing to do with your mistakes is to learn from them. Even if you fall or fail you must get up, dust yourself off, and try again. Believe in yourself.

Surround Yourself with Positive People and Positive Thoughts

Look for people who will encourage, uplift and affirm you. Be positive yourself, and give others the respect, dignity, and encouragement they deserve. Do not refer to yourself in a negative manner. If you constantly put yourself down, others will also. As someone once said, "Do not build a case against yourself."

Remember God Loves You Very Much

He loves and accepts you unconditionally, and His love for you will never change. He created you for a reason. He has a job that no one else can do as well as you. Go out today, and do that job in service to others, and do so in the Name of Jesus Christ.

Remember, there are no special formulas or pills that can "give" you a healthy self-esteem. Do not expect it to be developed overnight either. You must nurture it inside yourself day by day. Don't lose hope; with God on your side, you will make it.

Prayer: Dear God, thank You for making me the way I am. Help me to love myself. Today I say, along with the Psalmist, "I praise You because I am fearfully and wonderfully made; Your works are wonderful, I know that full well." Jesus, thank You for dying for me—that makes me very

valuable to You. Help me to use those gifts and talents You've given me, to reach out to others. I praise You for what You are, and what You are making of me. In Your precious Name. Amen.

Thought: We forfeit three-fourths of ourselves in order to be like other people.
—Arthur Schopenhauer

1 Thessalonians 5:11—Wherefore comfort ourselves together, and edify one another, even as also ye do.

37
Encouraging Other Nurses

We all need encouragement. It is as essential to our well-being as the need for water, food, and air. Deep down in all of us is the basic need to be loved and approved, to be liked and appreciated. An encouragement does all of these things for us. I cannot stress enough just how vital an encouragement is to a person. Celeste Holm, the actress, once said, "We live by encouragement and die without it—slowly, sadly and angrily."

The dictionary defines encouragement as "the act of inspiring with courage and hope." I like Donald Bubna's (*Encouraging People*) definition: "To come alongside another with a view toward helping in whatever way the person needs help."

Encouragement is not hard to give and it costs nothing to offer, yet it is one of the most difficult things for a lot of people to give to others. Three of these reasons are: a critical spirit, an unhealthy spirit of competition, and jealousy.

A Critical Spirit

Some people have the feeling that they must find something wrong with everything and everyone they encounter. They enter a room and all they see is that the drapes are hung wrong, the paint is awful, the carpet is dirty, the furniture is cheap and doesn't match. They meet a person and all they see are the terrible hair, the figure that is out of shape, the scars, the physical handicap, or the mistakes he has made. They don't take the time to look beyond the physical inadequacies, to see what that room or that person has to offer. They focus only on the negative; and they are so busy being occupied with the negative, they are unable to "see" the positive attributes.

An Unhealthy Spirit of Competition

Our competitive spirit sometimes restricts us from encouraging others as we should. In an unhealthy spirit of competition, our goal is to work harder than everyone else, get more money, become more popular, win more awards, achieve more recognition, power and influence, and climb the highest level of the administrative ladder. In order to do this we must step on other nurses, at times even our best friends, simply because we have the urgent need to beat out anyone else who seems to be ahead of us. Usually the tactics used include verbal attacks like slander, gossip and lies, withholding well-deserved compliments, and doing everything else within our power to disgrace that person.

A healthy spirit of competition is not bad; in fact, the Bible encourages this type of competition, but when our goal is to win at all costs, even if it means stepping on the heads of other nurses to get to the top, this is wrong.

Jealousy

Jealousy is also another reason why we do not encourage each other. The "green-eyed monster" clouds our perception and causes us to come up with devious ways to belittle the one who is the object of our jealousy. This might include humiliating them, or not encouraging them, or not giving them the credit that is due them. This too is wrong.

A great encourager or spirit-lifter has certain qualities. She is a good listener. She listens with her heart, without judging, condemning, correcting, lecturing, sermonizing or blaming. She is a sort of personal cheerleader, cheering you on to victory—"You can do it, you can do it, you can, you can!"

A great spirit-lifter is very sensitive to the feelings of others and recognizes their efforts and their improvements. She cooperates with other nurses instead of comparing or competing with them. She stimulates others instead of humiliating them, helping them to grow and reach higher heights, both in their lives and in their profession.

A spirit-lifter has a great sense of humor. She makes people laugh even when they want to cry. She accepts people as they are—warts and all, and uplifts them, displaying that she values them. She has a genuine concern for others and shows them respect and dignity. She also focuses on the positive things about people and accentuates these positives.

Of course, the ideal spirit-lifter does not exist, but several nurses I know and work with come very close to these qualities. They seem to uplift others by just being there, and they do so selflessly. They come alongside other nurses and support, affirm and encourage them by their words and deeds. You probably know nurses like that. What a blessing they are to the nursing profession!

It is important to note here that praise and encouragement are not the same. You praise a person by rewarding them on their achievements and for accomplishing some task. Encouragement is more than praise. It focuses on a person's assets, strengths, their efforts and improvements and other good things about them. It focuses on these positive things in order to help people build confidence, self-esteem, and self-worth. Encouragement enables people to believe in themselves.

Encouragement motivates and stimulates people. Other nurses are more likely to act the way we want them to, if we encourage instead of criticizing them for every little thing they do wrong. A little encouragement goes a long way. It makes people feel good about themselves, and when they do, they feel secure, accepted and adequate, and in this way, become more productive.

Encouragement also brings about growth in a person. It not only makes a person grow and flourish as an individual, it also enables them to grow into efficient nurses, working hard to deliver the best nursing possible to those placed in their care. Researchers say happy employees are more productive than those who are not happy at their jobs. Encouragement not only enhances productivity, it also brings out the very best in people. The following poem best describes what encouragement does for us:

> We blossom under praise
> Like flowers in sun and dew;
> We open, we reach, we grow.
> —Gerhard E. Frost

There are many other rewards for uplifting others. Blessings come to both the encourager and the person being encouraged. Encouragement alleviates depression and improves health. It uplifts the spirit, adds new dimensions to lives and brings about positive attitudes. It also creates beautiful thoughts and memories, not only for the person being encouraged, but also for the encourager, because as Proverbs 11:25 implies, you cannot help others without helping yourself. And, of course, the greatest reward of them all is to one day hear God say, "Well done, my good and faithful servant."

Ask yourself these questions: Do other nurses feel sure of themselves, and more valued when they are around you? Do you leave people feeling better about themselves as the result of their contact with you? Do other nurses look forward to working with you, and do they sign up for those shifts you work? Do they feel refreshed and nourished after they've spent a day with you? And do your coworkers come to you to be uplifted or "recharged"? If your answer to any of these questions is no, you probably need help in learning how to encourage others. The good news is encouragement skills can be learned and developed. Below are some suggestions on how to do this:

Love Unconditionally

Love is the key word here—love for God, yourself, and others. When we love people, it is easier to encourage them. We must not only love others because we expect them to give us something in return. We must love all people, regardless of race, creed or nationality. In order to love the way God wants us to, we must first love and accept ourselves as people made in God's image. This makes it easier to love and accept others and in turn to be able to encourage them to be better people. If you cannot accept yourself the way you are—the way God has created you to be—it will be very difficult to accept others, and love them unconditionally.

Be Willing to Sacrifice Yourself So That Others May Succeed

This is not an easy thing to do especially if you have an unhealthy competitive spirit, but this is what God expects us to do. As Christian nurses, our goal should be to encourage, affirm and support other nurses to become all they can be in the nursing profession. In this way we uplift them and ourselves also. Put others first. Help them and build them up to be better nurses. We must complement and edify each other so that together, we can give the best nursing care possible to our patients.

Encourage Others with Words

Words are powerful—they can make or break a person, build them up or tear them down. A careless "innocent" word can bring about degradation and low-esteem, and the pain could last a lifetime. On the other hand, a well-chosen, carefully thought out word can encourage a person and lead her to great achievements. Proverbs 25:11 tells us that words that are fitly spoken are like "apples of gold." A cheerful word is really good medicine.

Be sensitive to the feelings of others. Think, before you open your mouth! Remember, words can leave scars—scars that might never heal; so choose your words carefully. Your words must communicate to others, "I believe in you," "You are special," "I value your comments," or "I think you are great."

Words of encouragement can be either spoken or written. Spoken words of encouragement should be specific. For example,

"You have great leadership qualities," "You give the best massage," or "You are a great teacher." Also, be honest and sincere. People will see right through flattery. If you admire something about your co-workers, tell them; and do so in front of other nurses. Also tell them today. Don't wait until they are dead and gone. Words will be useless when they are dead.

Written words can also be a source of encouragement for others. Some people do not do very well with spoken encouragement. Writing also encourages. Even a brief note can communicate to another person that you value them and care about what happens to them. Use words that are warm, genuine and affirming, through cards, letters, recommendations and evaluations.

Encourage Others with Your Actions

As the saying goes, "Actions speak louder than words." You can encourage others without saying a word. You can do this by listening with the heart—not lecturing, condemning or sermonizing, but listening. When you listen with the heart, you are showing the other person that you are interested in her and about what happens in her life.

You can also encourage others by the way you look at them. A look can convey a lot. With a look you can communicate concern, love, disgust, joy, acceptance, hate, happiness, enthusiasm, approval, disapproval, and understanding. A look can also communicate, "I have time to listen to you," "I value what you have to say to me," "You are very important to me," or "At this moment, nothing is more important than you." It is of vital importance that we pay attention to our body language, facial expressions and direct eye contact when we encourage others.

Another way you can encourage others without saying a word, is by touch. Touch comes naturally to some and not others. The need for touch is universal. We are people, not machines—we need to touch other people.

Other actions that encourage include a smile, nod, humor, and selfless acts of hospitality like financial help, sharing, visitations, phone calls, positive feedback, and intercessory prayers.

Accentuate the Positive

You must propose in your heart daily to look for the good in people, and when you do, accentuate those assets and resources you see in them.

Possible areas include:

- <u>Physical appearance:</u> Hair, eyes, figure, clothes, jewelry, weight loss, makeup, accessories.
- <u>Mental or intellectual:</u> High IQ, knowledge in nursing, an ability to think fast on feet.
- <u>Personality:</u> Outgoing, dependable, friendly, strong-willed, determined.
- <u>Spiritual:</u> A good Christian, a spirit-lifter, a prayer warrior.
- <u>Performance:</u> A great blood draw, good IV start, great in emergencies.
- <u>Achievements:</u> Promotions, awards, citations.
- <u>Social:</u> Great relationship with coworkers, great with kids, great with patients and their families.
- <u>Leadership:</u> Fair, patient, supportive.
- <u>Emotional:</u> Stable, alert, great in emergencies.
- <u>Possessions:</u> great car, beautiful home, well-kept garden.
- <u>Talents and Gifts:</u> Culinary, arts and crafts, musical, athletics, artistic, generosity.

If you look with your heart, you will find something in every nurse to affirm her about. Today, go talent or resource hunting. You will be surprised at what you will find—hidden talents and treasures you never noticed before. When you find these talents and treasures, tap into them to enrich others and yourself.

You can even go one step further and help someone turn their liabilities and shortcomings into assets and strengths. For example, a bossy person could be a great leader, in charge and in control; a nosy person could be observant and inquisitive (two great assets for assessing patients); a talkative person could be friendly and informative, and great with patients and their families; or a fussy person could be a person who wants things to be exact and correct.

There are so many positive things to accentuate in a person! If you cannot find anything positive, maybe you are looking too close to the negatives you see in others, or you have not really "looked with the eyes of Jesus Christ." Remember, there is something good and right about <u>everyone</u>. Even a broken watch is right at least twice a day!

If you still can't find anything to encourage someone about, don't say anything. It is better to keep quiet than to say something that will cause low esteem and self-doubt in another person.

People need encouragement not only about their physical appearance, performance, achievements, assets and resources; they also need encouragement about their failures. Our encouragement will give them hope to try again. Let them know that we all have failed at one time or another, that mistakes are to help us learn, and that life is not always fair. Show them that you believe in them, that you will be there for them, and that you will be a shoulder to cry on, hug, or to just hold on to. Show them that you really care.

Look around you today. See that person who is going through a terrible divorce. Be the one who will uplift her spirit and affirm her. See the one that has a big decision to make, one that might affect her life in a big way. Maybe all she needs is the assurance that the decision she is making is the right one. See that one who is depressed because she's having a "bad hair" day. You be the one to cheer her up and "make her day." Or see that one who is discouraged and fed up with life. You be the one to give her the courage to "hang in there," and the hope to make it. Someone once said, "the best exercise for the heart is bending down and lifting up another person." How true!

Be an encourager and a spirit-lifter to your coworkers, and to your patients and their families. Always leave them a little better than you found them. Mike Murdock puts it this way: "You will only be remembered for two things: the problems you help solve or the ones you created." Let people remember you as an encourager and a spirit-lifter.

Prayer: Dear Lord, help me to be a spirit-lifter to those I live with and work with. Today, let me reach out to someone who is hurting, and comfort them. Let me use my lips to build up someone who might be going through discouragements and frustrations, and let me use my hands to uplift and support those who are down and out. Help me to emulate You, Lord, in my relationship with others. When they look at me, let them see a person they can come to, to feel better about themselves. Forgive me for those times I put others down by my words and my actions. From this day on, let me be a spirit-lifter. Amen.

Thought: Every day, by God's leading and enablement, each of us has it within his power to become a spirit-lifter.

—Virginia Whitman

Ephesians 6:19–20—And for me, that utterance may be given unto me, that I may open my mouth boldly, to make known the mystery of the gospel, for which I am an ambassador in bonds: that therein I may speak boldly, as I ought to speak.

38
Taking a Stand

We live in a banner-waving, cause-conscious generation. It appears that everywhere you turn, someone is "pushing" one cause or another. New Age believers are "pushing" the notion that one can find life, peace and salvation through some entity from "within" us and not from the Almighty God; environmental groups are warning about the depletion of the ozone layer; PETA is speaking against the unethical treatment of animals; gays and lesbians are fighting for their rights; feminists are emphasizing a woman's right to control her own body. The list goes on and on.

Surely no cause is more worthwhile for Christians than the cause of bringing Jesus Christ to a world that is hurting and dying. No cause is more desperately significant today than the need for Christ Jesus and His plan of salvation, for a world riddled with senseless violence, pain and disease.

How come we, who profess to be followers of the Living Christ, don't take a stand for Him?

There are several reasons why Christians don't take a stand for Christ. One of those reasons is guilt. When there are unconfessed sins in our lives, we are hindered from taking a stand for Jesus Christ as we ought to.

Another reason is fear: fear of what people will think or say about us. We think other people's impressions of us are more important than God's opinion. We are terrified of conflict and of "invading other people's privacy."

Shame and embarrassment are also reasons we don't like to

take a stand for Christ. We don't want to be known as "religious fanatics." We act as if we are ashamed of Jesus Christ and what He stands for. We would rather identify with the popular and worldly crowd than with Jesus Christ and Christian values.

Some don't take a stand for Christian values because of the lack of knowledge about certain biblical truths. They don't know what to say to back up what they believe in, and therefore don't say anything when the opportunity arises to take a stand for Jesus Christ.

Another reason why some people don't take a stand for Christian values is due to just plain laziness. They are not sensitive to the spiritual needs of those around them and are busy with the cares of the world. For them, standing up for Christian values takes too much time and effort.

Two of the best examples of believers taking stands for what they believed in are found in the book of Daniel. Chapter 3 tells about three young men who refused to serve the King's gods, or worship the golden image he had set up. Shadrach, Meshach and Abednego took a stand for God, and were willing to go into the fiery furnace rather than disobey God.

In chapter 6, Daniel was placed in the lion's den for praying and making supplications before God. He knew that taking that unpopular stand meant disobeying the royal statute of the King, and he was aware of the consequences of that disobedience, but that did not deter him. He obeyed God rather than man.

These men believed in their hearts that God's laws were indeed greater and more important than man's laws. They also believed that if they took a stand for God's laws, He would deliver them from harm. Their faith in God and His promises gave them the courage to take a stand for what they believed was right.

Through it all, God never left their side. He was there with them (as He had promised), in the fiery furnace, and in the lion's den, and He delivered them from harm. Their decisions to stand up for Him brought others (nonbelievers) to the Living God.

Taking a stand today may not be as dramatic as being thrown into a fiery furnace or facing vicious lions. It may not be as honorable as standing before a gang of hostile thugs as David Wilkerson did in *The Cross and the Switchblade*.

Taking a stand may be as simple as saying no to a dirty or racist joke while your colleagues look at you as if you were from another planet.

It may mean speaking up during coffee break and saying, "I believe abortion is wrong because the Bible says so," while the rest of the nurses look at you as if you are an idiot.

It may mean having to share your faith with a group of people who aren't very open or sympathetic to the cause of Jesus Christ.

It may mean speaking out for Christian values and family values, while the rest of the nurses snicker or call you a religious fanatic.

Or it may mean saying to another nurse, "I am sorry, but I can't take part in that."

It isn't very easy or even comfortable to stand alone. Taking a stand means having to take risks. Georgie Ann Geyer, a news correspondent, describes risk taking as "risking your popularity by taking a genuinely unpopular stand." It means risking your popularity, your career, your best friends, your family, and yes, even your life, to do what you believe to be the right thing in the eyes of God Almighty.

Taking a stand means stepping out in faith—faith in a God that others might not believe even exists.

In this day and age, when violence, hatred, and confusion seem to be the norm, and peace appears to be unattainable, God is calling on those of us who profess to be born-again Christians, to take a stand and let our voices be heard. We need to speak out for Jesus Christ and His truths.

We must be His voice—His voice to the brokenhearted, the downcast, the discouraged, and to those who are hurting. His voice to the people we care for, and to those we work with. His voice to the sick and dying world. <u>We must be His voice.</u>

Below are important guidelines to use when taking a stand for what you believe in.

Live Morally Right

Take a close look at your life. Confess your sins daily and ask God's forgiveness. Be honest with yourself. Allow the Holy Spirit to search your heart and to disclose to you areas which need changing or improving. Get rid of those sins that hinder our testimony and hinder our usefulness as Christians. Only after we let God straighten our own lives, will we be able to confront others effectively with the Word of God.

Be Firm and Courageous

Paul admonishes us in 1 Corinthians 15:58, "... be ye steadfast, unmovable, always abounding in the work of the Lord, forasmuch as ye know that your labor is not in vain in the Lord." Allow the Holy Spirit to give you the courage and the boldness to speak up for the truth, and to stand firm. If what you believe goes hand in hand with God's values, He will provide the strength needed to take that stand.

Study the Word of God

This will prepare you about what to say when you do take a stand. Read the Bible daily and memorize portions to use when it comes time to stand up and defend what you believe in. Allow the Holy Spirit to minister to you daily through the Word.

Be Aware of God's Presence

When we take a stand for Christian values, God does not just leave us there alone to take the rap. He has promised to be there, leading and guiding us. He has also promised to deliver us from the consequences of taking a stand on His behalf. He has promised to be there in our "fiery furnaces" and in our "lion's dens."

Love the Lord

When you truly love a person, you want to defend him every chance you get. If you love Jesus Christ, you will do everything within your power to defend Him and obey Him, even if that means having to give up your popularity, career, family and friends, and even your life if need be.

When You Take a Stand, Be Gentle and Patient

When people disagree with us we often get angry and defensive. We raise our voice, get red in the face, and the veins stand up on our neck. All these things are not necessary because truth carries its own force. The truth, backed by the Word of God, carries its own weight. Our job is to take a stand and do so gently and patiently. Leave the rest to God.

In this world filled with strife and torn with stress and tension, God is calling Christian nurses to stand up and let their voices be heard. We must emphasize the things that really count, and one of those things is the need for a personal relationship with Jesus Christ.

Don't be ashamed of Jesus Christ and what He stands for. Jesus tells us in Luke 9:26, "For whosoever shall be ashamed of me and of my words, of him shall the Son of man be ashamed, when he shall come in his own glory, and in his Father's, and of the holy angels." I don't want Jesus to be ashamed of me when I stand before Him that day, do you? Of course not.

Don't be a "closet Christian." Come out, take a stand! Let the world know you are a follower of Jesus Christ, and that you are not afraid or ashamed to say so.

Prayer: Lord, help me to speak boldly for what I know is right in Your sight. Please take away anything in my life that will hinder me from taking a stand for You. Forgive my sins and take away my feelings of fear, shame, and embarrassment. Instill in me a boldness for conveying the truths of Christ Jesus. Holy Spirit, teach me daily to study

the Word, so that when I do take a stand, I will be able to back it with sound Gospel. Help me to constantly be aware of Your presence in my life. Thank You for loving me. Amen.

Thought: I reckon him a Christian indeed who is not ashamed of the Gospel, or a shame to it.

—Matthew Henry

Matthew 9:37–38—Then saith he unto his disciples, The harvest truly is plenteous, but the labourers are few; Pray ye therefore the Lord of the harvest, that he will send forth laborers into his harvest.

39
Sharing Our Faith

The other day, a lady stopped by my house to sell cosmetics. She didn't start with her lotions, nail polishes, or sweet smelling perfumes; instead she spoke to me about glamour and beauty, looking good and feeling great, self-esteem, and how these liquids, cremes and powders could transform me into a "new" me.

She was a great saleswoman. By the time she left, she had my check of $90.00 for a bunch of cosmetics I truly believed would make me glamorous and beautiful. She had created in me the felt need for change, improvement, glamour and beauty, and in doing so, had sold her products.

As Christian nurses we have an obligation to "sell" Jesus to the people we meet—to our patients, their friends and families, our own families and coworkers. Like that saleswoman we must create in them the need for change and improvement in their lives: peace, intense joy, forgiveness of sins, unconditional love, and the continued presence of our Heavenly Father, among many other benefits.

"How can I sell Jesus?" you might ask. You can do so by sharing your faith with others. You can do so by becoming a soul-winner.

Contrary to popular belief, soul-winning is not for everyone. Before you start to disagree with me, give me a few minutes to explain myself. There are certain prerequisites for those of us who want to be soul-winners for Christ. They are simple requirements, but important ones, no less.

First, you must be born again. In order to efficiently lead others to Christ the Savior, He must be Lord over your life. In other words, you must know the Way to show the way to others.

You should have a working knowledge of the Gospel. The Bible is the spiritual food which nourishes us and prepares us for our call to duty. It tells us what to say and, with the power of the Holy Spirit, can stir up the person we want to lead to Christ.

Another requirement is falling in love daily with Jesus Christ. When you love someone dearly, you can't help talking about him. Likewise, if you truly love Jesus Christ, you would love to tell others about Him and about His saving grace.

You must also love people enough to long for their salvation. When you love someone, you want the very best for them, and surely, their salvation is one of the best things you can wish for them. If you truly love people, there should be a longing in your heart to lead them to Jesus. If you truly love and care about people, you will have the desire to see them saved, and on their way to heaven.

It is also important to pray daily, taking unsaved people to the Lord in prayer so that God can prepare their hearts for Christ's message of love and salvation. Also pray that the Holy Spirit ministers to these people.

Lastly, you must be Spirit-filled. Acts 1:8 tells us that Jesus told His disciples, "But ye shall receive power, after that the Holy Ghost is come upon you: and ye shall be witnesses unto me both in Jerusalem, and in all Judea, and in Samaria, and unto the uttermost part of the earth."

The Holy Spirit brings us boldness, radiance, joy, enthusiasm, confidence and courage to witness to even the most difficult person. He strengthens, energizes and empowers us for effective service. In short, He gives us the tools for our outreach to others.

You might be asking the question, "What's in it for me?" There are rewards for those of us who win souls for Jesus Christ.

We cause heaven to erupt in rejoicing and celebration when we win one soul for Jesus Christ. Luke 15:10 attests to that. It states: "Likewise, I say unto you, there is joy in the presence of the angels of God over one sinner that repenteth." Isn't it a great thing that you and I are capable of causing such intense feelings of joy and celebration, by leading even one person to Christ?

Secondly, it gives us a sense of fulfillment that we are being used by God Almighty to carry out His mission. What a privilege it is to be called God's ambassador! There is nothing more satisfying. What an honor to be chosen by God to speak on His behalf.

What amazes me even more is the fact that God can use simple, insignificant people like you and me, to do such a great and important job as ambassadors for Him. Friends, this is honor indeed!

God has rewards for soul-winners. In addition to vast benefits including eternal life (which we are assured when we become born again), we will receive other rewards like blessings (Psalm 115:12), honor (John 12:26), inheritance (Colossians 3:24) and a crown of glory.

I don't want to leave you with the notion that everything about soul-winning is peachy. There are costs to winning souls for Christ.

Winning souls takes time and energy. It takes the time you could be watching TV, knitting, skiing, or doing things you enjoy. It takes energy that could be spent for your own purposes, instead of studying, praying and preparing for soul-winning. In short, it complicates your life, but wouldn't you rather spend the time and energy and invest them in reaching out to those who would otherwise die in their sins if it weren't for your pointing them to Jesus Christ?

In the business of soul-winning you stand the risk of embarrassment, rejection and even persecution. It is embarrassing when people think you are a fanatic, or just plain crazy because of your belief in Christ, or because of your system of values. It hurts deeply when people reject you or refuse to believe that Jesus Christ is for real, or that He really saves lives. Worst of all it is difficult when you are persecuted because you want to follow Christ.

In America we are blessed that we don't often see the types of religious persecution others suffer in some countries, even today. All over the world, Christians are persecuted daily for trying to bring lost and lonely souls to Jesus Christ.

Soul-winning may also cost you money. It may mean spending your money for Christian books, tracts, badges, greeting cards, buttons, Bibles, etc., to reach others for Christ. It might mean sending money to help others (i.e. churches and missionaries) to reach others for Christ. Or it might cost you a loss in salary.

Soul-winning requires time, energy and money, and involves the risk of rejection, embarrassment and even persecution, but it is worth it, many times over. "The closer you look, the more you see that the rewards are high and the costs relatively low, especially when we understand that ultimately they're not costs at all. They're investments that pay permanent dividends."[1]

There are several ways to share your faith. Below are four ways to witness, along with some suggestions or examples. They are: silent witnessing, opportunistic witnessing, invitational witnessing, and personal testimonies.

Silent Witnessing

You can witness this way by being "salt," or by letting your light shine wherever you are—at home, church or at work. Examples of this type of witnessing are:

1. Living a clean and morally decent life at *all* times.
2. Speaking up against evil.
3. Taking a stand for Christian values.
4. Giving your time, energy, money and service to help uplift others. You can do this by:

- <u>Cards.</u> Inspirational cards that encourage and uplift, cards with scriptures, Christmas and Easter cards celebrating Jesus, cards praising and thanking God for his blessings, get-well cards that let others know how much they mean to Jesus, cards that give religious meanings of names, etc.
- Plaques and badges that express Christian values. Keep

in mind that your objective is not to manipulate others, but rather to inspire.

1. Praying openly at lunch or during breaks.

Opportunistic Witnessing

This type of witnessing involves creating opportunities to talk about Jesus Christ to others. Examples:

1. Conversations that lead to Him.
2. Counting your blessings and openly thanking the Lord for providing these blessings.
3. Pointing out the good things about this world and the fact that it is God's handiwork.
4. Exalting God in your daily life.
5. Expressing joy, and when asked why you are so happy, giving Jesus the credit.
6. Looking for signs that show that the person is religiously inclined, for example, a cross, pictures of angels, a Bible, a pastor visiting, or visitors from the church, etc.
7. Asking questions like: "Is there someone praying for you?" "Can I pray for you?" "Can we pray together?"
8. Letting people see you reading Christian literature like the *Journal of Christian Nursing, Moody Magazine, Focus on the Family,* etc., or letting them see you as you listen to Christian radio.

Invitational Witnessing

This type of witnessing involves inviting others (patients and their families, or coworkers) to church, Christian programs, and other activities that enlighten and uplift our Lord Jesus Christ.

Personal Testimonies

This is a realistic appraisal of what Christ has done in your life. It must be realistic, specific and precise and should include:

1. What your life was like before Christ entered it and became your Lord and Savior.
2. How you came to know him.
3. What is happening now in your life because of His presence.

There will be different reactions to your witnessing. Some will refuse Jesus Christ and His plan of salvation. Others will mock or ridicule you. But on the other hand some will accept Him and still others will accept the challenge to share their faith with others. In this way, the Gospel will spread.

You may not be able to cross the ocean and go to far away places like India or Pakistan, or go deep into the African jungles to share your faith with people who are lost and in darkness.

You don't have to go to the primitive people of New Guinea or to the poor lost souls of South America to be a missionary for Jesus Christ. You don't have to risk your life or the lives of your loved ones in war-torn Bosnia or other troubled areas in the world in order to be a servant of God. You can be a missionary right here in your own country, your state, your workplace.

I am from Africa (a place sometimes referred to as the "dark continent"), a place thousands of people have gone to, to bring the light to a world of darkness, but I see people right here in America, who are also in darkness and in dire need of the light that only Jesus Christ can give.

Jesus told His disciples, "The harvest truly is plenteous, but the laborers are few; Pray ye therefore the Lord of the harvest that he will send forth laborers into his harvest" (Matthew 9:37–38). This is also our call to duty as Christian nurses, by the Lord of the harvest.

There are many people out there who desperately need to know Jesus in a personal way, yet hundreds of thousands are going to hell right now because we don't want to take the time to tell them about His plan of salvation. There's a lot of work to be done and as Christian nurses, we have an obligation to bring those people in contact with Jesus Christ before it's too late.

As we reach out to share our faith with others, there are three important things to keep in mind.

First, there is no better witness to the reality of the power and love of our Lord Jesus Christ than a Christian nurse whose daily life and conduct bears out his or her profession of salvation in Him. Talk is cheap, as the familiar saying goes. Sharing your faith is not enough; you must also practice or live what you preach. Actions truly speak louder than words.

Billy Graham puts it beautifully: "Sermons which are seen are often more effective than those which are heard."

Secondly, it is not enough that we offer our patients and their families information about Jesus Christ and His saving grace. We must first deal with their physical and emotional needs, then ease in the need for spiritual wellness. We must not neglect their physical and emotional needs. This is all part of care giving. We must first meet these needs, then introduce them to the Jesus Christ you and I know, trust, and believe in. In this way, we minister to the whole person.

Lastly, if someone agrees to accept Christ, and wants you to pray with them, remember that the prayer doesn't have to be long or elaborate; the intent of the heart is what is important. Be sure to touch the person and hold her hands as you pray, and tell her about the Great Physician, His control over lives, and changes His love brings to empty lives.

Spread the News

If you truly believe you have the good news, spread it around. Spread it to the pregnant teenager who's thinking about abortion, and the lonely teenager contemplating suicide. Spread it to your coworker going through family crisis, and the family of the critically ill child. Spread it to the woman dying from breast cancer and the person living with HIV. Spread it to the infertile couple desperately seeking a child, and to the elderly desperately looking for someone to talk to. Spread it to the one who is hurting, discouraged, and disillusioned, and to the one who believes all hope is gone.

Spread it around,
Spread the Good News around.

<u>Prayer:</u> Lord Jesus, wherever I go today, and whosoever I come across, make me a true witness for You. There are many that are hurting and lonely, who need that special touch from You. May they see Your light in me and come to know You personally. Let me live in such a way that people will "see" my sermons. Amen.

<u>Thought:</u> In order to share our faith with others, we must catch a glimpse of their hearts—their motivations, hurts, needs, and purposes. We must begin to see them as the Lord Jesus sees them.

—Roberta Hromas

Note

1. Bill Hybels and Mark Mittelberg, *Becoming a Contagious Christian* (Grand Rapids, MI: Zondervan Publishing House, 1994), p. 38.

Ephesians 3:7—Whereof I was made a minister, according to the gift of the grace of God given unto me by the effectual working of his power.

40
Tools of the Trade

As we go about our ministry of service to others, there are special tools that we use to carry out our duties as Christian nurses. This chapter deals with three of these tools that are essential for reaching out to others in the name of Jesus Christ. They are a touch, a smile, and humor.

Touch

There is no question about it, human touch is crucially important to our very existence. Deep down inside all of us is the need to be touched by other human beings. A hug, a hand on the shoulder or arm, a handshake, or a pat on the back—all these actions help us to relate to other people in a special way. It is indeed a pity that not many people utilize these actions to reach out to others.

There are reasons why we don't like to touch or be touched. The #1 reason is fear fear of what people will think. People are afraid that others will think they are homosexual if they touch or are touched. Also, with the increase in sexual harassment, incest, rape, and child molestations, people are afraid that their touch will be misinterpreted for an inappropriate gesture. Some people feel very uncomfortable when touched by others. They feel that when others touch them, their space is being invaded. Fear is almost always a tool of Satan. He uses fear in order to put a wedge in our relationships with others. He uses fear so that we can become isolated and alone in our own tiny world, not touching or being touched by other human beings. This is not in God's plan for our lives.

Another reason why we don't like to touch or be touched by others is because some of us have a feeling of superiority—not wanting to be touched by "untouchables." (It is important to note here that people who are sick or less fortunate than we are, are sometimes considered "untouchables.") Our Lord Jesus Christ loved to touch others, especially those considered "untouchables." He reached out with love and compassion to these people and healed them physically, emotionally and most importantly, spiritually. As Christians we too must emulate Jesus, and reach out to these people, and touch them.

Healthy and appropriate touching is correlated with empathy, love, compassion, warmth, genuine concern for others, positive self-esteem, encouragement, trust and a sense of relationship. A touch sends out messages: "It is all right to touch me," "I think you're okay," "I like you," or "I am interested in you." Appropriate touching enhances emotional health and affirms others. It is a pity that so many people miss out on the valuable qualities that a healthy and appropriate touch brings.

Famed marriage and family therapist Virginia Satir once said: "We all need about eight hugs a day to feel healthy." I strongly agree with her. We must communicate to our patients and their families that we truly care for them and their needs, and we must do so by touching them in a special way. I encourage you today to reach out to your patients—hug them, put your arms around their shoulders or on their arms, or pat them on their backs. It doesn't matter which one you do—just do it!

Smile

We know that it takes 26 muscles to frown, but only five muscles to smile. It's plain and simple, being constantly sad and grumpy causes wrinkles! Unfortunately many of us walk about every day, just asking for wrinkles!

Smiling doesn't take much effort, but we sometimes allow

our negative feelings and other things to affect our actions. Some feel that they have to be happy in order to smile, or that things have to be working out well in their lives before they can smile. As Christians, we are encouraged to have joy in our hearts constantly, and a smile lets the world see a glimpse of what we feel inside. If we say we have the joy of the Lord in our hearts, the world must see it on our faces. Someone has said, "The smile on your face is the light in the window that tells people that you are at home."

A smile affects the sender and the receiver. It uplifts all it touches; it breaks the ice and sets the mind at ease. A smile also makes friends, because it truly is the shortest distance between two people. A smile lets the world experience the joy you say you feel inside.

A smile is contagious; but unlike the common cold or other bacteria and viruses, a smile is a great thing to spread around, because it benefits everyone it touches.

A smile is a valuable tool to use in reaching out to our patients and their families. Below is a poem I read in a book some months ago. It gives a good description of what a smile is:

> A smile is cheer to you and me
> The cost is nothing—it's given free;
> It comforts the weary—gladdens the sad,
> Consoles those in trouble—good or bad.
> To rich and poor, beggar or thief,
> It's free to all of any belief;
> A natural gesture of young and old
> Cheers the faint, disarms the bold;
> Unlike most blessing for which we pray
> It's one thing we keep when we give it away.
>
> — Author unknown

Use a smile to reach out to your patients today.

Humor

I strongly believe that God has a marvelous sense of humor, don't you? Or else why would He allow hospital gowns that open at the back; or infants who wait until you remove their diapers, then aim straight for your face; or the elderly patient who tries to "gum" you.

Humor brings laughter and laughter uplifts people and makes them happy. It brings joy, lightens the load, creates a good mood, releases stress, and diverts attention from problems, pain, hurts, etc. What a powerful tool to be used in caregiving!

Humor and laughter create sociability, and establish relationships. Humor usually doesn't exclude others; instead, it includes people and makes them laugh together. In short, it unites people.

Some say it heals—a sort of "merry medicine." Proverbs 17:22 states, "A merry heart doeth good like a medicine: but a broken spirit drieth the bones." Studies have shown that laughter helps the body in several ways:

1. It aids the entire respiratory system by cleaning it out.
2. It exercises the heart, thorax, abdomen, lungs and diaphragm.
3. It supplies six times as much oxygen to the body as a deep breath.
4. It stimulates the endocrine system and aids in the digestion of food.

It is very important to remember that humor can be used as a tool or a weapon. Just like any good thing created by God, Satan can cause us to use this beautiful tool as a weapon to hurt others. Below are ways humor can be used as either a tool or a weapon:

Tool	Weapon
to uplift	to degrade
to teach	to belittle
to amuse	to abuse
to relieve stress	to bring about stress
to unite	to divide
to elevate	to tear down
to help	to hurt
to make friends	to make enemies
supportive	derogatory
involves all	excludes some people
can be delightful	can be crude and inappropriate
laughing with others	laughing at others

Joel Goodman gives a good example of the difference between laughing with people and laughing at them: "Laughing with someone is going for the jocular vein, and laughing at others is going for the jugular vein."

It is important to think of others before you make a joke. We must use humor with integrity and care. This involves being sensitive to others' feelings. Be careful to use humor as a tool to help your patients to heal, instead of as a weapon.

When we use humor with our patients, we are in a way helping them to heal faster and in this way, we minister to the whole person. Laughter is truly the best medicine!

Some believe that for a joke to be funny or accepted, it must be filthy or a racial, cultural, or sexist stereotype. Let us be reminded that as Christians we must use our words to build up and uplift others, and to glorify God.

I have come across several jokes that are clean and also humorous. Below are some of my favorites. I am unable to list each author of these jokes because many of the authors are unknown, and some of the jokes have been attributed to more than one author.

The young mother was telling the visitor about her child:

"He's eating solids now. You know—keys, bits of newspapers, crayons, pencils."

A small town is where everyone knows whose check is good and whose husband isn't.

Some people cause happiness where they go; others when they go.

A bright eye indicates curiosity; a black eye, too much.

Before you put too much faith in a rabbit's foot for luck, remember it didn't do much for the rabbit.

Ulcers are what you get from mountain-climbing over mole hills.

A vacation consists of 2 weeks which are 2 short, after which you are 2 tired 2 return 2 work, and 2 broke not 2.

Nothing improves a person's driving like the sudden discovery of a police car parked on the corner of the street.

Social tact is making your visitors feel at home, even though you wish they were.

We spend the first 12 months of our children's lives teaching them to walk and talk, and the next 12 years telling them to sit down and shut up.

Favorite Jingles

Late to bed and early to rise
Makes a nurse baggy under her eyes!

Don't pass cars on curve or hill
If cops don't get you, the mortician will!

It's easy to tell sinner from saint.
Sinner is always the one you ain't!

A little flattery now and then
Makes husbands out of single men.

The boss is a person
You should never get smart with;
You might be the one
He can easily part with.

Some Bloopers Found in Various Church Bulletins

The Little Mother's Club holds its regular meeting Tuesday at 4 p.m. All those who wish to become Little Mothers, please see the pastor in his study after the service.

Tonight's sermon: "What is Hell?" Come early and listen to our choir practicing!

This being Easter Sunday, we will ask Mrs. Peters to come forward and lay an egg on the altar.

This afternoon there will be meetings in the south and north ends of the church. Children will be baptized at both ends!

Don't let worry kill you, let the church help.

Ladies of the church have cast-off clothing of every kind, and they can be seen in the church basement on Friday afternoons! Everyone is welcome.

On Sunday, a special collection will be taken to defray the expense of the new carpet. All wishing to do something on the carpet, please come forward and get a piece of paper.

Wednesday, June 10th, the Ladies Liturgy Society will meet. Mrs. Jones will sing, "Put Me in My Little Bed," accompanied by the Pastor.

Thursday night—potluck supper. Prayer and medication to follow.

For those of you who have children and don't know it, we have a nursery downstairs.

More Jokes

It is a strong but mathematical fact that when a 17-year-old boy borrows the family car, he can, in one night, subtract five years from the life of the car and add them to the age of his father.

Out of the mouth of babes often come remarks their parents should never have said in the first place.

A sign on a wall somewhere in Europe: "God is dead—Nietzsche"; underneath had been added "Nietzsche is dead—God."

Criticism is the one thing that most of us think is more blessed to give than to receive.

The forbidden fruit is responsible for many a bad jam.

Going to church doesn't make you a Christian any more than going to a garage makes you an automobile.

Constructive criticism is when I criticize you. Destructive criticism is when you criticize me.

A mosquito is like a kid. When silent, it's up to something!

Drive carefully! Remember—it's not only a car that can be recalled by its maker!

Sign In Department Store

Wonderful Bargains in Shirts for Men with Sixteen and Seventeen Necks.

Sign in Dry Cleaners

Pants Pressed in Rear During Alterations

Sign in Gas Station with Adjoining restaurant

Eat Here, Get Gas.

<u>Prayer:</u> **Jesus, thank You for Your great examples on healing. You know how to heal the whole person. Lord, teach me to do likewise. Help me today, to reach out to the people You've placed in my care. Let me emulate Your love, compassion and Your concern for them, with every fiber of my being. Let me smile, use humor, and reach out and touch them in a way that will bring glory to Your name. Amen.**

<u>Thought:</u> You are God's gift to the world. Do all you can do to make it a better place.

—Alma Kern

Part Five

Specific Devotionals

There are certain topics and issues that are unique to different types of nursing. In this section, inspirational devotions are developed around these topics and issues which feature personal meditations filled with Scripture, life-changing insights, and practical applications, designed to help the nurse grow in her walk with the Lord.

> Ecclesiastes 12:13–14—Let us hear the conclusion of the whole matter: Fear God, and keep his commandments: for this is the whole duty of man. For God shall bring every work into judgment, with every secret thing, whether it be good, or whether it be evil.

John 3:3—Jesus answered and said unto him, verily, verily, I say unto thee, except a man be born again, he cannot see the Kingdom of God.

41
Newborn Nursing

There is certainly no joy like the one seen on the faces of a man and wife as they hold their brand-new baby in their arms for the first time. For the last nine months, they have waited patiently for this day and for the arrival of this precious being. Finally that day is here. In their arms is the most beautiful baby in the world, with her cute button nose, tiny mouth and dainty fingers and toes. Even with the "cone head" and the bruises and abrasions, they still believe she is the most beautiful baby in the world.

The journey from embryo to fetus and then to a baby is an intricate and wonderful process designed by the Almighty Himself.

From the exact moment the sperm penetrates the egg, a new life begins, and the fertilized egg begins its slow journey down the fallopian tube and into the uterus, where it will find a suitable environment that will protect, care for, and nourish it until it is able to survive on its own. Then the day arrives when the mother's cervix dilates with contractions, and the tiny, precious individual enters the world stark naked, helpless, confused, defenseless, and sometimes a bit battered from delivery—but a gift that will bring intense joy and happiness for the parents, other relatives and friends.

When I look at the birth of this newborn, I am reminded of the new birth that is mentioned in the third chapter of the Book of John. This passage tells us about a conversation between Nicodemus and Jesus Christ.

Nicodemus was a member of the Sanhedrin (a group of men who were the religious ruling body of Israel and were considered the highest authority on the Scriptures). Nicodemus had come to Jesus at night, seeking answers to questions that were troubling him. He wanted to know if Jesus was really what He claimed to be. Nicodemus saw that there was something in the life of Jesus Christ (something lacking in his own life) that set Him apart from other religious leaders, and Nicodemus wanted to know what that "something" was.

Jesus looked at him and told him that he must be born again in order to have the chance of eternal life. Jesus had looked at the heart of Nicodemus and knew that more than anything else, Nicodemus needed a rebirth. His position, riches and vast knowledge of the Scriptures could not qualify him for salvation and eternal life. There was only one way he could qualify—he had to be born again.

The term "born again" is almost two thousand years old. To be born again is to come to know God personally and become a member of His family. This happens when you acknowledge the fact that Jesus Christ is who He says He is, confess your sins, repent, place your faith in Him, and receive Him as your Lord and Savior. This personal relationship with Jesus Christ is the beginning of a new life under God's control. This process brings with it a changed life—with changed affections, changed will, and a changed purpose for living. You become a new creature. This spiritual transformation is called being born again.

There are striking similarities between a physical birth and a spiritual birth. First, in both cases pain is involved. In the physical birth the mother has pain with contractions and pushing. Of course, since epidural is being widely used now, some of this pain is subdued during contractions, episiotomy or the repair of the episiotomy. In the spiritual birth, Jesus Christ, the Son of God, bore pain which now makes it possible for us to be born again. He was beaten, and a crown of thorns placed on His head, nails driven into His hands and feet, and He was hung to die on the cross, and then His side was pierced. Oh, what terrible pain He must have suffered!

There are other similarities. In the physical birth, the baby is born naked and alone. Even twins are not born at the exact same time. When you become born again, you do so by yourself.

No one can make that decision for you. Even if your father is a minister, or your mother a deaconess, this doesn't make you a born-again Christian. You must appear before God yourself, and when you confess your sins to Him, you stand before Him alone and naked for His scrutiny.

In the physical birth, when the baby is born, everyone including the doctor, nurses and the parents await the first cry. This lets them know the baby is alive and okay. Likewise, the new, born-again Christian needs to say his first words. This is the public confession proclaiming his new relationship with God, and his membership into the family. He needs to tell others about his new life. This is a sign that will let others know he is now born again (Matthew 10:32, Romans 10:9, 1 John 4:15).

In the physical birth, the baby is helpless and totally dependent on his parents. Likewise the baby in Christ is helpless and has to depend on Jesus for spiritual survival.

The birth of a baby brings joy to the parents, family and friends. The spiritual birth also brings about jubilance on earth and in heaven. The Bible tells us in Luke 15:7 that likewise there shall be joy in heaven over one sinner that repents.

The moment a baby is born he becomes a part of a family, with all the benefits that come with that family. The moment we become born-again, we become part of God's family, with all the benefits of the child of the King. The Bible tells us that we have a new inheritance—we become a joint heir with Jesus Christ Himself (Romans 8:14–17)!

A baby is born at a specific time—minute, hour, day and year. We are also born again at a specific time. In the physical birth, the baby is no longer just a baby boy or baby girl. He or she is now given a name such as Shawn, Mary, Abby, Matthew. When we are born again, we are called born-again Christians.

The baby needs milk, a food that is high in protein, fat and carbohydrates, otherwise he would be malnourished, leading to stunted growth or susceptibility to various diseases. Failure to thrive or malnutrition can be detrimental to the baby's physical health. The spiritual newborn also needs spiritual milk, which includes daily prayer time, Bible study, and constant fellowship with other Christians; otherwise spiritually, his growth is stunted and he becomes highly susceptible to all kinds of spiritual diseases. Two Peter 3:18 states that we are expected to "grow in grace and knowledge of our Lord and Savior Jesus Christ."

Lastly, the baby has its first bath, when the blood, vernix and meconium are washed from the baby's body and he is dressed in beautiful warm clothes. Likewise, the spiritual newborn is baptized in water. Mark 16:16 states, "He that believeth and is baptized shall be saved; but he that believeth not shall be damned."

All these and many more show the striking similarities between these two types of births, but there are two major differences between them. First, the physical birth has an end result that is temporary, but the spiritual birth is for eternity. Christ Jesus tells us in John 3:16 that whoever believes in Him shall "not perish, but have everlasting life."

Secondly, the physical delivery is usually in a hospital, in a controlled environment, with a special bed, good light and sterile equipment used for this procedure. God's "delivery room," where a person becomes born again, can be anywhere he is willing to turn his life over to Jesus. You can become born again anywhere—in your bedroom, in a church or a hospital bed, on a plane, or on a street. You can also become a born-again Christian at any time, <u>even this minute.</u> You don't have to wait for nine months. Now is the accepted time, now is the day of salvation (2 Corinthians 6:2).

Let me ask you this—today, can you say without reservation that you are born again? If your answer is "Yes," you have the assurance of eternal life through Jesus Christ. If your answer is "No," the good news is that it is not too late to become a born-again Christian. Won't you say yes to Jesus Christ today? Give your life to Jesus right now, and become a member of His family, enjoying all the benefits that come with being a child of God. <u>Do so today.</u> No one knows the future. Today might be the last chance you have to accept Jesus Christ. Below is a simple way to give your life to Him.

1. Realize these facts:
    God loves you very much, enough to give His only begotten Son so that "Whoever believeth in Him should not perish, but have everlasting life" (John 3:16).
    Even though God loves You, He still hates sin, because it separates us from Him.
    You are a sinner. "For all have sinned and come short of the glory of God" (Romans 3:23). "If we say we have not sinned, we make Him a liar, and His word is not in us" (1 John 1:10).
    There is a penalty for sin. "For the wages of sin is death, but the gift of God is eternal life through Jesus Christ our Lord" (Romans 6:23).
    Christ already paid the penalty for your sins. "But God commendeth His love toward us, in that while we were yet sinners Christ died for us" (Romans 5:8).
    Salvation is free to all. "For by grace are ye saved through faith, and that not of yourselves: it is the gift of God: Not of works, lest any man should boast" (Ephesians 2:8–9). Nothing you do in your own power or strength can save you. You cannot buy your salvation either; it is a gift from God to you.
2. Repent of your sins. "Except ye repent ye shall all likewise perish" (Luke 13:3). It is not enough to feel sorry or guilty for your sins. "If we confess our sins He is faithful and just to forgive us our sins, and to cleanse us from all unrighteousness" (1 John 1:9). No matter how big you think your sins are, if you honestly admit your guilt, He will forgive you. And His forgiveness is complete.
3. Receive Jesus Christ as Lord and Savior. "But as many as received Him, to them gave He power to become the sons of God, even to them that believe on His name" (John 1:12). Right now Jesus is knocking on the door of your heart. He will never force His way in, you

must make a decision to let Him in. If you want to be born again, repeat this prayer:

Jesus, I know I am a sinner, and I believe only You can save me. Forgive the sins I have committed in words, thoughts and deeds. Thank You for dying on the cross for me. Right now, I surrender my life to You and accept You as Lord and Savior. Fill me with Your Holy Spirit. Thank You for saving me. In Your precious Name. Amen.

4. <u>You become a born-again Christian the moment you receive Jesus Christ.</u> You may or may not feel a drastic change in your life right away, but remember, the new birth is not a feeling. It is receiving Jesus Christ by faith. You can now say with assurance, "I have received Jesus as my Lord and Savior. I now have eternal life!"

5. <u>Confess Christ Jesus publicly.</u> Jesus said, "Whosoever therefore shall confess me before men, him will I confess also before my Father which is in heaven" (Matthew 10:32). Tell others about how you met Jesus and about the changes He has brought to your life.

6. <u>As a newborn Christian, you need spiritual "milk"</u> for growth and strength to fight Satan's darts. (Now that you are born again, he is not happy!)

7. The spiritual "milk" consists of:

<u>Bible study.</u> Get a Bible and read it daily. Saturate yourself with it and memorize portions of it so that you will be prepared when Satan shows his face. (Believe me, he will—after all, he just lost you to Jesus Christ.)

<u>Learning how to pray</u> (see chapter 34).

<u>Finding fellowship with other Christians.</u> Look for a Bible-believing Church and a Bible study group or prayer group.

As you feed daily on the spiritual food, you will become more and more aware of God's presence and guidance in your life. <u>Wel-</u>

come to God's family! If you just accepted Jesus Christ as your Lord and Savior, I would like to know about your decision. Write to me at the address below.

Kay Marie Bani
P.O. Box 3852
Littleton, Colorado 80161-3852

<u>Prayer:</u> **My Lord and Savior, thank You for my salvation. Thank You also for the assurance of eternal life with You. Holy Spirit, give me the boldness to tell everybody I meet today, that I am a born-again Christian. As I go about my job, let me emulate Your love and compassion as I reach out to those who are placed in my care. I am truly blessed to be chosen by You, to be Your ambassador in my workplace. Thank You again that my sins are forgiven, and I am on my way to heaven. I pray this prayer in Your precious Name. Amen.**

<u>Thought:</u>
    Life is uncertain,
    Death is sure;
    Sin is the cause,
    Christ the cure.

—Author Unknown

Romans 8:14•15—For as many as are led by the Spirit of God, they are the sons of God. For ye have not received the spirit of bondage again to fear; but ye have received the Spirit of adoption, whereby we cry, Abba, Father.

42
Family Care Nursing

"He looks just like his daddy." "She has her mother's hair." "He has the Logan ears." "He has his father's eyes." These are familiar statements that are made after the birth of a baby. Nothing brings greater joy to a daddy than being told that his newborn son (or daughter) looks just like him. From his parents, the baby inherits his color, stature, hair texture, race, certain abnormalities such as extra digits, certain disease conditions and other genetic disorders.

When growing up, the child learns most of what he knows by watching others (particularly his parents) and modeling himself after them. There is no question that the greatest incentive to the development of a child's character comes from a modeled behavior rather than from specific instructions.

A child learns to walk, eat with a spoon and dress himself by example. And he learns to speak by his parents' example. Just as the child learns from their good examples, he also learns—sad to say—from their bad examples. If you hear a kid using vulgar, sexist or racist words and wonder where on earth he got such language, wait a while and listen to his parents talk! As a familiar saying goes, the fruit doesn't fall far from the tree.

It is indeed incredible how powerful a father's behavior or example can be upon his children. When a boy puts on his father's shoes, or when a little girl tries on her mom's hat and earrings and uses her lipstick, they are both trying to model a significant person in their life. They want to resemble their parents.

As Christians we also want to look like our Heavenly Father. If we say we are children of God, we must exhibit attributes that are Christ-like. These attributes include the fruits of the Spirit, a controlled tongue, obedience to God, forgiveness, and a consistent pattern of Christian living. These attributes make us resemble our Heavenly Father. When others look at us they must be able to say, "He looks just like his Daddy."

When you think of your father, what kinds of memories, feelings or images do you summon up? Perhaps, you remember a stern, unfeeling, unloving, and unforgiving father who was more concerned about his car or watching sports on TV, and was never available to you.

Maybe you remember a daddy who deserted you and your siblings, and never took the time to provide for you or even inquired about your life. The number of "deadbeat" fathers continues to grow today, even among Christian families.

Perhaps you had a father who molested you in ways that were despicable and you've had to carry those terrible images with you all these years.

Or maybe you remember a daddy who was affectionate, kind and uplifting, willing to spend quality time with you and who had a great sense of humor, and made his family his number one priority.

Whether you had a father like those in the first three descriptions, or one like the last, you probably carry with you memories that affected your life long after you left home. You remember the negative feelings of violence, betrayal, angry words, put-downs, rejections and neglect, but you also remember the positive images of love, acceptance, happiness, joyful moments, and a sense of togetherness. These feelings and memories help shape your future. Too bad a lot of fathers do not realize the influence their conduct and example have on the lives of their children!

Now, let me tell you about our Heavenly Father. He loves us very much and His love is unconditional. Good or bad, tall or short, black or white—we are precious to Him. He wants the very best for us; that is why He is not willing that even one of His children should perish in sin. That is why He sent His precious Son to die in our place. John 13:16 reminds us of that love: "For God so loved the world, that he gave his only begotten Son, that whosoever believeth in him should not perish, but have everlasting life." God wants us to not only have salvation, He also wants us to have everlasting life through His Son, Jesus Christ.

Our Father wants to spend time with us. He wants to have a close, intimate relationship with us. And when we are hurting, confused or lonely, He is there, waiting to pull us into His bosom, just as a mother gathers a child who has been hurt, wipes the tears, kisses the pain away, and lets him know that it's going to be okay. God the Father wants to enfold us into His great big arms and wipe away our tears and make everything fine again. He is a haven we can run to, when the world becomes cruel, unrelenting, and painful. No matter how old we are, we still have that "childlike" feeling inside when pain, trouble and disappointments come. We still need our Daddy to comfort and sustain us. We still need that tenderness that only He can give.

But God our Father gives us even more. When we are depressed, weak, tired and weighed down by the cares of this world, He gives us the strength and courage to cope with the stresses of life.

God did not promise that there will never be hard times in our lives. He never promised that there will never be discouragements, disappointments, frustrations and pain. He lets us know that He will never desert us or leave us to suffer alone. He promises His presence with us through every valley. His very presence gives us comfort, courage, and strength. How good it is to know that He is _always_ near, looking out for us.

Like a good father, God also disciplines His children. When we break His laws or disobey His Word, we have to bear the consequences of our disobedience, yet He loves us despite our sinful actions.

Let us remember this—we have a Father in heaven who loves and cares for us, and wants to meet our every need. The Word of God admonishes us to not worry or be anxious about what we will eat, what we will drink, or what kind of clothing we will wear. Our Father <u>knows</u> we need these things, and He is willing to provide them for us. We only need to call out to Him. If He takes care of the flowers and provides for the birds, how much more will He do for us. After all, He sacrificed His own Son in our place. There is nothing He will not do for you or me. When we cry "Abba, Father," we touch a chord in Him, and He reaches out and helps us.

Let us also be reminded that if we call ourselves children of God, we must walk, dress, talk and act like children of the Heavenly Father. We must be a mirror image of our Father. When others look at us they must be able to see a God that is loving, kind, forgiving, merciful, and caring.

<u>Prayer:</u> My Heavenly Father, thank You for being my comfort, my strength and my courage. Thank You for loving me even though I let You down by the things I say, think and do. Thank You for the times You've had to discipline me when I've disobeyed Your Word. Thank You for not giving up on me. Most of all, thank You for sending Your Son Jesus Christ to die on the cross for my salvation. Amen.

<u>Thought:</u> Have you ever noticed how children want to be just like their parents when they are young, nothing like their parents when they are teens, and then they become <u>just</u> like their parents when they become adults?

—Charles Williams

Leviticus 19:32—Thou shalt rise up before the hoary head, and honor the face of the old man, and fear thy God: I am the Lord.

43
Nursing of the Elderly

For those nurses who care for elderly patients, it takes a special kind of gift to reach out to those people and care for their physical and emotional problems. It also takes a special kind of Christian nurse to minister to them spiritually.

There are certain important facts about aging that we must know if we are to be the best nurses for our elderly patients.

The older population is steadily increasing. Scientists tell us that by the year 2030, about 65 million Americans will be 65 years or older. This means that approximately 20 percent of Americans will be over 65. Life expectancy has been extended due to modern medical technology, improved health care delivery, and a trend towards healthy living such as good eating habits, exercise and the cessation of smoking.

Old age is inevitable. If we are blessed with long life, we will all be old one day. It is part of God's plan for our lives. As the years go by, we get older. No matter how hard we try to beat old age by using makeup, dyeing the hair, facelifts, etc., old age is inevitable. It creeps up on us all slowly but surely.

The great commission commands us to go into the world and teach all nations about Jesus Christ. This call to ministry is to all who call themselves born-again Christians. Our ministry should be to everyone, including the elderly. As Christian nurses, we must minister to the elderly patients who have been placed in our care, but in order to give them the best spiritual care, we must first understand what it means to be an elderly person. Let's look at some of the limitations and benefits of aging.

Limitations

Some of the limitations are physical. There is a waning of some of the senses. Usually the most apparent are the sense of hearing and the sense of sight. Hearing aids and thick glasses become a way of life. In addition, there is the limitation of mobility, poor circulating in the extremities, and loss of sexual desire. The gray hair, sluggish GI system, and reduced sense of taste, all add to a sense of loss, but there are many other kinds of losses also.

There is significant loss of the social role. In a society where work defines self-worth, the loss of a job (through retirement) might mean to some a loss of value and productivity. To some, it might mean a loss of avenues to express their power and authority, or a loss of their part in decision-making. To still others, it might mean an economic loss due to no regular income, no support from family members, little support from social security, and no retirement pension or savings.

Another limitation is the loss of independence. For years they've been considered valuable, resourceful people whom others depended on for livelihood; now they have to rely on others for almost everything. When they become sick, it becomes even worse because they are unable to care for themselves. The humiliation of this dependency is sometimes too much for them to handle. In addition, the elderly are very vulnerable to people who like to take advantage of older people.

Lastly, there is a loss of acquaintances. More and more people their age are passing away. Their spouses, former classmates, coworkers, and friends are dying, and this loss, along with the other losses and limitations, only leads to loneliness, fear, grief, and a sense of insecurity. In spite of these losses and limitations, which Arthur H. Beckers (*Ministry to Older Persons*) calls "a thousand little deaths," there are also benefits to aging.

Benefits

Old age is usually referred to as the "Golden Age." Old age is a time of peace and relaxation. There is no need to prove oneself, therefore, there is a sense of freedom to be oneself. Also, because the elderly person is retired and has a lot of spare time on her hands, she can now make new friends and spend more time with her children and grandchildren. The spare time also makes it possible for her to serve others and to enjoy the beauty of nature and many other blessings.

Old age also brings with it maturity and wisdom (Job 12:12). The elderly can teach the younger generation a thing or two. Their wisdom comes from the experiences (both good and bad) of their lifetime. We can learn a lot from them.

Lastly, old age brings with it an openness to accept Jesus Christ and the things of God. This is usually a time of soul searching. I have found out that it is a lot easier to witness to the elderly because they are more open to the Word. This openness towards God is a great advantage because it makes it easier to reach out to these people with the Gospel.

The elderly might be frail, but they are not worthless or useless individuals who are just taking up space in this universe. They are valuable people who can contribute greatly to society. We must remember this as we minister to these people. The poet Henry Wadsworth Longfellow put it well when he wrote:

> What then? Shall we sit idly down and say
> The night hath come; it is no longer day?
> The night hath not yet come; we are not quite
> Cut off from labor by the failing light;
> Something remains for us to do or dare;
> Even the oldest tree some fruit may bear,
> For age is opportunity no less
> Than Youth itself, though in another dress.
> And as the evening twilight fades away
> The sky is filled with stars, invisible by day.

Now that we know the limitations and benefits of aging, let us discuss what elderly people need from us.

The Bible tells us to honor and respect the elderly (Leviticus 19:32, Proverbs 23:22, 1 Timothy 5:1–2). They deserve to be treated with dignity and they need our praise, recognition, encouragement, and a part in decision-making. They need association with others, security, orientation, creativity and assurance. They need better health care, more transportation facilities, better housing, better access to healthy meals, companionship, and much, much more. These are needs we are all entitled to, but the elderly need them even more.

More than anything else, we need to give our elderly patients hope, not only for early recovery from the hospital, but also for eternal life through Jesus Christ.

It is not enough that we tell these people about God, and about salvation through Jesus Christ; we must do so with honor, respect, and dignity. We must let them know how valuable they are, especially to Jesus Christ. Let us be reminded that even though the body is frail and old, these people are made in God's image, and therefore deserve the very best care that we can offer them physically, emotionally and spiritually.

Reach out today to an elderly person and let her know how much Jesus loves and cares for her.

Prayer: Lord, thank You for choosing me as an ambassador to my patients. Help me to be the "salt" that seasons their bland lives and the "light" in this world of loneliness and darkness. When they look at me, let them see a life that exemplifies Your love and compassion. I pray that You will root out everything in my life that will hinder my call of ministry to my patients. Thank You, Lord, for my salvation and the chance of eternal life with You. These things I ask in Your most precious Name. Amen.

Thought: Nearly two-thirds of all the greatest deeds ever performed by human beings—the victories in battle, the greatest books, the greatest pictures and statues—have been accomplished after the age of sixty.

—Albert Edward Wiggam

Luke 9:2—And he sent them to preach the kingdom of God, and to heal the sick.

44
Emergency Room Nursing

The emergency room is usually busy with patients in serious conditions needing immediate care; therefore, it is sometimes very difficult to share our faith with our patients. However, even in this busy, noisy, fast-paced atmosphere, we can still reach out to our patients and let them know that Jesus Christ loves them.

Man is more than a physical or emotional being. He is also spiritual, so if our goal is to treat the whole person, we must be concerned about our patients' physical, emotional and spiritual conditions. When we look at our patients, we should see them as people who are not only in need of IVs, bandages, X rays or pain pills, but also as individuals in need of Jesus Christ. Luke 9:2 tells us that Jesus sent His disciples to "preach the Kingdom of God, and to heal the sick." Healing the sick involves treating our patients physically and emotionally. Telling them about the Kingdom of God is caring for them spiritually.

Let us look at an example of how Jesus Christ Himself heals people. Mark, chapter 2, relates a story about four friends who heard about Jesus and His healing power, and tried to get their friend, who was sick with palsy, into the crowded room in order to see Jesus and be healed. To do this they had to open the roof to let their friend into the room. When Jesus saw their faith, He said to the sick man, "Son, thy sins be forgiven thee." Even before healing the man physically, Jesus knew that more than anything, this man needed to be healed spiritually. Later He healed the man physically. He healed the whole man.

Jesus was concerned about that man's spiritual condition just as He is concerned about people's spiritual condition today.

If we want to emulate Him we must also be concerned about the spiritual condition of our patients. We must look at our patients with the eyes of Jesus Christ.

Below are suggestions on how to witness to your patients in the emergency room:

1. <u>Strive to be a consistent Christian.</u> Live up to what you profess to be. Let others "see" your Christianity, not only hear you say you are a Christian.

Be a Christian at all times, not only on Sunday or during prayer meetings. At work, home or play, our lives should exemplify the life of Jesus Christ. One benefit of living a Christian life at your workplace is when patients request a Christian nurse, or someone to pray with them, your coworker will point to you and say, "She's a Christian nurse."

Take a stand for Jesus Christ and for Christian values. Glorify God in public and let others see and hear you pray in the open. Do not be ashamed of Jesus Christ. Identify yourself as a born-again Christian. Come out of the closet, and let the world know that you are a Christian and that you are proud of it.

To identify yourself as a Christian involves certain things. You must have unconditional love for people. You must also surround yourself with things that glorify Jesus Christ. One of the marks of a genuine Christian is a spirit-controlled tongue. Use your tongue to uplift others and glorify God. Do not use filthy language, gossip and put others down, but encourage and build others up, and give God the glory for things that have happened in your life. Also let them see the "joy of the Lord" in your face. Joy will set you apart from other nurses, and people will want to know why you are the way you are. This gives you a chance to tell them about Jesus.

2. <u>Carry Christian literature around with you.</u> Try to find tracts or small cards with words of inspiration that tell about Christian values and how to be saved. I usually buy tracts and cards from the Christian bookstore and hand these out to my patients at appropriate times. These don't cost a lot, and they fit perfectly in the pockets of scrubs. If a patient is in severe pain or in

a very critical condition, it might not be an appropriate time to have him read, but let him know you are leaving him something to read when he feels better.
3. <u>Pray with your patient</u> if he allows you to. Remember, you cannot force him to pray if he doesn't want to. First suggest it to him and when he agrees, hold his hands and say a short prayer for him. Also include him on your daily prayer list.
4. <u>Do not ignore the patient's physical and emotional care.</u> Be reminded that our object is to treat the whole person.

Sometimes, it takes only a few minutes to share your faith with your patients and their families. Be sure to make good use of those few precious minutes—somebody's soul might depend on it. And if you lead even one person to the Lord, it will be worth it.

Jesus has called us not only to heal or cure the sick, but also to preach the Kingdom of God. He has placed you in that specific emergency room for a purpose. Your being there is not by chance. He wants to use you as a channel for His love and compassion to those who are placed in your care. As you go about your job, keep this fact in mind: Whatsoever you do today for the least of these people, you're doing it for Jesus Christ.

Prayer: My Heavenly Father, thank You so much for calling me to Your ministry in the emergency room. Help me to live in such a manner that people will be able to identify me as a born-again Christian. May I truly live what I preach. Holy Spirit, prepare the hearts of people I will meet today—let them be willing to listen to the Word. When I witness to them, teach me the right things to say. May Your name be glorified through me. Thank You for loving me. Amen.

Thought:
> Do others know from how we act
> At home, at work, at play
> That we have Jesus in our heart
> And live for Him each day?
> —Dennis J. DeHaan

Matthew 23:11–12—But he that is greater among you shall be your servant. And whosoever shall exalt himself shall be abased; and he that shall humble himself shall be exalted.

45
The Nurse in Administration

"It's so lonely at the top," goes the chorus of a familiar song. Being a leader is one of the loneliest jobs an individual can undertake. Leadership is not glamorous, and it comes with a price. It might mean working long hours, sometimes unappreciated, frequently alone. It appears like you are never off duty. As soon as you think you have a few minutes for yourself, there comes the ring of the phone with someone at the other end wanting you to solve a problem or make an important decision.

When an individual climbs to the top, he or she leaves so much behind—close friendships, self, and at times peace of mind, but leadership can also be rewarding and fulfilling. Christian nurses in leadership positions are blessed—they have a great model to follow—our Lord Jesus Christ.

Jesus Christ was the ideal leader. First of all He was a qualified leader. He didn't leap into leadership. Even though He was Christ, the Son of God, He spent 30 years of His life preparing and training for three years' work.

Secondly, He was a humble servant. In fact, He regarded servanthood as the prerequisite to leadership. He was the most humble of all men. He displayed this humility by getting on His knees and washing the feet of His disciples. Washing feet was one of the lowliest jobs in those days. It was a job done by a house slave, yet Christ the King did it to prove a point: to be a leader we have to have the heart of a servant.

Thirdly, He studied the Scriptures daily and preached the Gospel. Even though He was God, He still turned to the Scriptures for knowledge and guidance—He included God the Father in His decision making.

Fourthly, Jesus looked past people's faults, and saw their needs. He was sensitive to their needs and genuinely cared about how people felt and what happened to them.

Lastly, Christ had a vision. When He left heaven to come to earth, He knew He was coming to die for our sins. His vision was to save souls, and nothing could deter Him from that goal—not even death!

There is much we can learn from the life of Jesus Christ. As Christian nurses in administration, we must continually yearn to learn more and keep abreast of new trends and discoveries in our career. We must use every available opportunity to enhance and increase our knowledge, ability and efficiency in leadership.

We must be Spirit-filled (led by the Spirit), and guided by God. He should be a major part of our decision-making. When faced with difficult and critical decisions, we must ask ourselves, "What would Jesus do if He were in my place?" We must ask the Holy Spirit to give us sound reasoning, clear thinking and judgment, and constantly seek mature counsel of trusted and reliable people.

Like Jesus Christ, we must be humble servants. This involves losing self and becoming self-sacrificing. We must be willing to sacrifice ourselves so that others might succeed. This is not an easy thing to do, but it is required of us. Their success is also our success. We must help others discover and channel their gifts and talents for the good of the people who are placed in our care. We must also be willing to give ourselves up and over entirely (without reservation or compromise) to the perfect will of Jesus Christ in order to be useful in His service.

A great leader must be sensitive to the needs of subordinates. We must treat individuals as unique human beings and not as objects without feelings. We should never fit everyone in the same mold. We must be peacemakers, creating climates of harmony instead of discord, and maintaining fellowship and cohesiveness among our employees. This involves being careful about how, when, and where to confront individuals, being fair, and serving as an encourager, affirmer, and a cheerleader.

As leaders, we must be able to listen not only with our ears, but also with our hearts. We must help others to feel worthwhile. Although self-esteem is defined as how one feels about his own worth, a person usually builds these feelings from the messages he receives from others, especially those in leadership positions. We must inspire and infuse our subordinates with an exalting spirit of enthusiasm for caregiving.

We must also learn to effectively delegate responsibilities not only to the most capable, but also to those who need the experience. No one believed in delegating responsibilities more than Jesus Christ. He knew the importance of giving His disciples the responsibilities of becoming future leaders themselves, after He was gone.

Delegation has numerous advantages. It relieves us from doing all the work ourselves and gives us the chance to be available for other chores. It supports workers to develop confidence in problem-solving, prepares them for greater responsibilities, and helps build trust and cooperation. Lastly, it encourages more adequate teamwork.

A great leader is never a "Lone Ranger." She needs a team. She needs a network of nurses and other employees pulling together to a common goal—giving the best care for our patients. We must maintain a close relationship with our employees, seek wise counsel from trusted friends, and look to the team for input on decision-making.

Lastly, like our Lord and Savior, we must have a vision, knowing where we are going, and the means of getting there. This involves faithfulness, determination, strong willpower, and a willingness to work hard and long in order to see that vision accomplished. As the familiar phrase goes, "If you aim at nothing, you will hit it every time!" We must become visionaries if we expect great things to happen in leadership.

You might be saying about now that these qualifications seem like a tall order, but be reminded that leadership comes with a price. Not everyone is qualified to be a leader. God has placed us in that leadership position for a reason. We have been called by Him to be His ambassadors.

Let us not be discouraged and quit. There will always be

pressure, stressful situations and trials. The Bible tells us to expect these things in 1 Peter 4:12. These tests or trials are necessary because they keep us humble so that we may not feel it was our power that put us in such high position. They also increase God's power in us. In 2 Corinthians 12:10b, Paul tells us: "For when I am weak, then am I strong." In our weaknesses, He is strong. Our trials also produce perseverance and maturity (James 1:2–4).

We might never receive awards or earthly crowns for the work we do. Others might not see or appreciate the hard work we do while our colleagues are sleeping or out enjoying themselves, but there is One who sees <u>everything</u> we do, and He will reward us one day.

We must be prepared to receive criticisms. People will question our motives and methods of doing things or making decisions. They might cast doubts on our authority as leaders. People are often fickle. They sing our praises one day, and the following day they might curse or criticize us. Sometimes these criticisms are motivated by fear, uncertainty or jealousy. Let us be reminded that not everyone will agree with us on every issue. There will always be individuals who will complain, grumble, backbite and gripe about one thing or another.

Remember, Jesus also faced critics. Here was a man who was without sin—a Perfect Person, yet people found something wrong with Him. The Pharisees and scribes constantly criticized Him and found fault with everything He said or did. His enduring patience should be an example to us when we are criticized, or when our decisions are questioned.

And when it gets lonely at the top, let us be reminded of the presence of God. He promises to never leave us or forsake us. We are not alone in our service to others. We must rely on Him for guidance, direction and companionship.

<u>Prayer:</u> Father, thank You for placing me in this position of leadership. Help me to serve humbly, putting You and the needs of others first. Mold me, teach me and lead me so that I can be the best I can be. I give You the glory and honor in my service to others. Holy Spirit, fill me with

Your power and boldness, and allow me to genuinely reach out with my heart to those I work with. Lord, in me, let them see a leader who truly portrays You in everything I do and say. When I am lonely and discouraged, help me to look to You for strength, direction and companionship. Amen.

Thought: If you wish to be a leader, you will be frustrated, for very few people wish to be led. If you aim to be a servant, you will never be frustrated.

—Frank F. Warren

Ephesians 4:11–12—And he gave some, apostles; and some, prophets; and some, evangelists; and some, pastors and teachers; for the perfecting of the saints, for the work of the ministry, for the edifying of the body of Christ.

46
The Nursing Educator

If you ask who I think is the greatest teacher, I will say without reservation, it has to be Jesus Christ. He was a master teacher. He knew the significance of teaching; teaching people was of such importance to Jesus that He included it as part of the great commission: to go heal, go teach and go preach.

As Christian educators, we are called to carry out this commission, where we live, work or play. Our profession is our ministry to our students and their families, and we must model our teaching career after that of Jesus Christ, the greatest teacher of them all. His profound teachings informed, inspired, motivated and stimulated people, and caused many to change their lives for the better.

As Henry Adams appropriately put it, "A teacher affects eternity; no one can tell where his influence stops." How very true. Even though teachers don't get paid nearly enough for their vast contributions, the students they tutor go on to become great nurses, holding offices, healing and caring for people and helping others live better and resourceful lives. The influence of these teachers continues long after their students leave the classrooms.

We all can remember one or two teachers in our lifetime, who made major impacts in our lives. They were people who believed in their pupils, and loved and cared enough for them, that they went over and above their call to bring out the very best in their students.

My father, Johma Massaquoi, was such a teacher. It's been several years since his death, but his students still tell me what a great teacher he was and what an influence he had on their lives. They have gone on with their lives, yet the knowledge he gave them continues to this day.

I also had teachers who made huge impacts on my life. One of these was a Peace Corps volunteer named Alfredo Pons and the other was my literature teacher in high school, Lillian Bartholemew. I still remember how these teachers believed in me and made me feel important. There was something else they did— they made learning a joy for me. I could hardly wait to get to their classes. To this day, I believe that they helped shape my life as a writer. I am presently searching for these teachers to let them know that I appreciate them.

Great teachers have certain qualifications that stand out. Three of these are scholarship, enthusiasm, and a great sense of humor.

A teacher must know what she is teaching. She must study and keep abreast of the latest in nursing. The Christian educator must also have a working knowledge of the Bible so that she can be prepared to witness to her students and her colleagues. She must not only be concerned with the physical and emotional aspects of the lives of her students, but also the spiritual condition of their lives.

Enthusiasm is another quality that makes a great educator. Synonyms of enthusiasm include fire, spirit, force, zeal, eagerness, optimism, feeling, hope and power. A great teacher must bring out these feelings in her students. This enthusiasm transforms and changes lives and beliefs. It motivates and captivates imaginations and in this way encourages students to be the very best they can be. This enthusiasm will touch a chord in the lives of students and make a difference in their lives.

A great sense of humor is another asset for the educator. It puts students at ease, releases tension, and helps them to open up in order to exhibit their potential. Again, it brings out the best in them.

Let us follow the example of Jesus Christ, "who saw people not as they were but as they could be with His help and guidance."[1] As Christian educators we must look beyond that scared, insecure and clumsy nursing student and see the potential for a great nurse—maybe another Florence Nightingale.

Like Jesus Christ we must inform, inspire and motivate our students. We must stimulate them to action and provide incentives to them for accepting Christ as Lord and Savior, and for living pure lives. It is important that we develop students who will become efficient nurses, but it is more important that we develop nursing students who are saved, forgiven, Spirit-filled and on their way to heaven. Let's not forget that these future nurses will be caring for people who also need to know the Lord. Our career is our ministry. Along with nursing education we must preach and teach the Gospel. Most importantly, our own lives must mirror that of Jesus Christ. Let us live in such a manner that our students and colleagues will see a living Christ in us, and come to respect and adore Him, and want to know Him personally. Let us remember that most of the lessons these students will absorb will be from watching what we do rather than what we say. People would rather <u>see</u> a Christian than hear one.

Let us keep in mind that we will be called to give an account of our lives before the Almighty God.

We must not be discouraged if our present salary is disproportionate to the type of work we do, or if people are not giving us the thanks and appreciation we deserve. Galatians 6:9 tells us: "And let us not be weary in well-doing: for in due season we shall reap, if we faint not." This is a promise! God sees everything we do, and He will repay us.

Our Lord has chosen us to be His special ambassadors in the classrooms, labs and clinical areas. He has set us apart to bring glory to His name. Let us get serious about spreading the gospel of Jesus Christ to a world that is dying spiritually.

Prayer: Heavenly Father, thank You for calling me to be Your ambassador in my classroom. Jesus, thank You for Your love which encourages me to be the best teacher I can be. Let me model my career after Your masterful examples. Holy Spirit, empower me with the boldness, confidence and courage to witness to even the most difficult

people I come across. Thank You for Your continued presence in my life. Amen.

Thoughts:

> The mediocre teacher tells,
> the good teacher explains,
> the superior teacher demonstrates
> the great teacher inspires.
>
> —Wm. Arthur Ward

> To teach is to learn.
>
> —Japanese proverb

Note

1. Jerry Stubblefield, *The Effective Minister of Education: A Comprehensive Handbook* (Nashvile, TN: Broadman and Holman Publishers, 1993), p. 167.

Revelation 21:4—And God shall wipe away all tears from their eyes; and there shall be no more death, neither sorrow, nor crying, neither shall there be any more pain: for the former things are passed away.

47
Working with HIV and AIDS Patients

How did he get it? Is he gay? Does he do drugs? These are all questions we ask when we are assigned a patient who is HIV positive or has AIDS; but is that the most important thing about that patient? Does it really matter now, how he got it? I think not. What is essential is that there is a sick and desperate individual who has come to us for the treatment of a fatal and infectious disease that is slowly sapping the very life out of him. Usually, by the time this person comes to us, this lethal and life-threatening illness has already taken its course.

AIDS (Acquired Immune Deficiency Syndrome) is a disease caused by the human immune deficiency virus (HIV), which impairs the immune system of an individual, resulting in a wide range of consequences, from asymptomatic conditions, to life-threatening opportunistic organisms like Pneumocystic carinii, and certain tumors such as multifocal Kaposi's sarcoma. AIDS is the terminal stage of this disease, when the individual who is infected can no longer control the organisms or the malignancies that rarely cause illness in people with competent immune systems.

AIDS was first described in the United States in 1981. At that time, it was generally known as GRID (gay-related immune deficiency syndrome), or "the gay man's disease." More and more doctors in New York and Los Angeles began noticing a strange phenomenon in homosexual men. Young and virile men were developing strange lesions and were dying from complications of illnesses that seldom cause sickness in healthy people. This brought about major concern to the doctors, but little from the rest of the population. It wasn't until 1985, when Rock Hudson died of AIDS, that people began to pay serious attention to this devastating illness.

The AIDS virus is 20 times smaller than the herpes virus, and about 450 times smaller than a sperm cell, yet this minute and deadly organism continues to cut short the lives of thousands at an alarming rate.

In the USA, an estimated 1 million people are infected with HIV; and as of 1995, approximately 350,000 AIDS-related cumulative deaths have occurred. Globally, an estimated 14 million people are infected with HIV. Projections also estimate that between 38 million and 108 million people will be infected by the year 2000. Of course, these projections do not take into account AIDS cases that are never diagnosed or reported.

People with AIDS suffer in numerous ways. First, they suffer the horrible physical effects of the terrible disease that has invaded their bodies. Symptoms include fever, significant weight loss (also called wasting syndrome), encephalopathy, recurrent bacterial pneumonia, PCP, Kaposi's sarcoma, invasive cervical cancer, TB, candidiasis, and toxoplasmosis of the brain, to name a few.

Secondly, people with AIDS suffer from the emotional and psychological effects of being stigmatized by people around them. Along with the stigma comes condemnation, desertion, and abandonment, not only by their families, friends and loved ones, but also by others they are in contact with.

Lastly, they suffer an economic impact. The cost of providing medical care and psychological services to AIDS patients is soaring, and most insurance companies refuse to insure these people. Losses also are incurred by disability, loss of jobs, and housing, and other discriminations.

As Christian nurses caring for patients with AIDS, we must be careful not to condemn these individuals when they are placed in our care. We must not add more pain, guilt, degradation and shame to people who are already suffering from this horrific illness, that is (in a way), a death sentence. These people do not need our pity, contempt, or condemnation. They need our love, compassion and support.

When we condemn these people, we break their spirit, weaken their faith, cause them to close their ears to the Gospel, and push them further and further away from Jesus Christ.

We must show them love, compassion and tolerance; give them hope, and point them toward Jesus. In this way, we emulate our Lord and Savior.

In the book of John, chapter 8, the Bible states that Pharisees and scribes brought a woman to Jesus who had been caught in the act of adultery, and they asked Him what to do with her. It was the law of Moses that a woman caught in adultery should be stoned to death. Jesus answered them and said, "He that is without sin among you, let him first cast a stone at her" (John 8:7)." The Word tells us that the men left one by one. They had been convicted by their own conscience.

We ought to remember this story the next time we want to condemn others for their sins.

As Christians, we often walk around with our gavels, condemning others for the sins we find in them, forgetting, of course, the sins in our own lives. Matthew 7:1 warns us against such act: "Judge not that ye be not judged." The Word goes on to tell us in Matthew 7:5, "Thou hypocrite, first cast out the beam out of thine own eye; and then shalt thou see clearly to cast out the mote out of thy brother's eye."

There might be more than just a mote in the other person's eye, and it might be charitable for you to want to help remove it for him, but Jesus sees it another way. He tells us to first consider the beam (which is much larger than a mote) in our own eye and remove it, then we can see better to remove the mote from our neighbor's eye.

Removing our own sins and faults has advantages. It doesn't only help us see better, it makes us free to venture out and help others to remove their own shortcomings, and also gives us the authority to criticize others, but based on the Word of God.

Being a Christian does not make us perfect. On the contrary, it makes us better able to see our own sins and faults, and to honestly turn these areas over to Jesus, who is the only One who can forgive and liberate us. Then and only then are we ready to assist others remove the problems in their lives.

When people with AIDS are placed in our care, we must remember Christ's compassion for people that others considered outcasts, untouchables and undesirables. <u>He looked beyond their faults and shortcomings and saw their needs.</u> We too must look beyond their problems and see individuals with needs—physical, emotional and spiritual needs, and try to meet these needs the way Jesus Christ would.

These people are sick, lonely, and in terrible pain. They need our friendship, support and hope. We must let them know that we truly care for them. All it might take is a shoulder to cry on, a hand to hold on to, a comforting word, a sympathetic ear, or a warm touch of another human being. Let's be reminded that AIDS is not spread by casual physical contact, or by hugging, touching or shaking hands. We should reach out to them with our hands and our hearts, and help make their present suffering more bearable.

And above all, let us tell them about Jesus Christ—an understanding and compassionate Savior, who knows and feels the pain and suffering they are going through. These individuals need to know that He listens when they cry out to Him. They need to know that when medical science offers no more hope, when families and loved ones abandon them, or when it appears that the whole world has deserted them, Jesus will still be there, waiting to love them and care for them. He has promised to <u>never</u> forsake them or fail them the way so many have. It was for people like this that He shed His Precious blood on the cross. These individuals need to know that!

As Christian nurses, we have been called to care for these people, regardless of the nature of their illness or the means by which they got it. With their discolored skins marked with multiple lesions, their wasted bodies, gaunt faces and sunken eyes, still they are made in God's image, and are therefore very valuable in His sight. Jesus Christ died for them, and He wants them to know that He cares greatly about what happens to them. <u>We must tell them about Jesus!</u>

The book of Revelation, chapter 21:4 tells us, "and God shall wipe all tears from their eyes; and there shall be no more death, neither sorrow, nor crying, neither shall there be any more pain: for the former things are passed away." People with AIDS need to know this wonderful promise of a better life. We might just be the only ray of hope they have for that life.

<u>Prayer:</u> **Father, thank You for placing _____ in my care. I realize the great responsibility You have given me to be Your ambassador in my workplace. Let me be an instrument used by You to reach out to him with love, compassion and hope. Let me be that beacon light that will lead him to You. Remind me daily that despite his illness, he is very valuable to You, and that You love him dearly. Thank You today for choosing me to be his nurse, and for being a part of Your healing team. I ask these things in Your Precious Name. Amen.**

<u>Thought:</u> The Son of God suffered unto death, not that people might not suffer, but that their suffering might be like His.
—George MacDonald

Isaiah 41:13—For I the Lord thy God will hold thy right hand, saying unto thee, Fear not; I will help thee.

48
The Nurse Who Is Out of a Job

Amy, a new graduate nurse, has passed the state board exams, and is anxiously looking for her first job. She knows a lot of nursing theory but has had very little experience with patients, except the hours spent on her clinical rotations. Most of the hospitals she has applied to require at least one year of experience with direct patient care.

Katie has been a registered nurse for about six years, and during this time has already had to change jobs three times. She is not satisfied with her present job. Stress, depression and burnout have slowly crept in, and the workplace has become intolerable for her. If she doesn't find another job soon, she doesn't know what she will do.

Julie was called to the head nurse's office and told that because of corporate downsizing and pending layoffs, the lactation department, where she works, has been eliminated, and the hospital can no longer use her. This has come as a complete surprise to Julie who has worked with this hospital for the past ten years.

Caroline is 55 years old. At 53, she had asked for and received an early retirement from the hospital she had worked for, for the last 25 years. Now she's having financial problems, so she's looking for a part-time job. She has applied to three hospitals already and has not heard from any so far.

These four nurses have one thing in common: they are going through a job crisis. Anyone who has been out of a job, or is dissatisfied with her present job, knows how devastating it can be. A job crisis is a serious reality for a lot of nurses, and can have major impacts in four areas: economic, emotional, social and spiritual.

Economic

A job crisis can mean a loss of regular income. When there are bills to pay, tuition due, piano and dance lessons to pay, mortgages, car payments, and other necessities, and there is no income to pay for these, the loss of financial stability and security can only add to anxiety and fear of what the future holds for the family.

Emotional

A job loss can cause anger and low self-esteem, in addition to anxiety and fear. Rumors of mergers, layoffs and downsizing do not help either, because they bring about widespread jitters, worrying and hopelessness, which usually lead to a lowered morale.

Social

A job crisis can also have serious and social impacts on an individual. It can rip a family apart, especially if there are no savings to fall back on. Most nurses I know are the sole providers for their family's financial needs, and the loss of a job can be nerve-wracking for everyone, including the children. But sometimes, if the family is strong, this crisis could draw them closer together.

Spiritual

A job loss can also have a spiritual impact on a person. The question is usually asked: "If God really cares for me, why is He allowing this to happen to me?" A job loss can either cause an individual to lose his faith in God, or it can cause one to draw to Him and become totally dependent upon Him for his every need.

Are you going through a job crisis today? Does it seem that nobody understands what you are going through? Are you facing financial troubles that seem more than you can bear? Let me assure you, there is hope. Below are some suggestions on how to cope at this time of uncertainty and anxiety.

Pray

At a time like this, draw closer to God and continue to pray. Tell Him what you want and ask Him to help you. Matthew 8:7 states, "Ask and it shall be given you; seek, and ye shall find; knock, and it shall be opened unto you." This is a promise from your Father in heaven. All you have to do is ask. Be specific, and tell Him exactly what you want. James 5:16 tells us, "The effectual fervent prayer of a righteous man availeth much." Live a righteous life and God will do His part.

Jesus tells us in Matthew 6:31–33 to stop worrying about what we (and our families) will eat, drink or wear. Our Heavenly Father already knows we need these things. Jesus goes on to tell us to first seek His kingdom and His righteousness, and all these things will be given to us. This is a promise you can take to the bank.

Consider Your Options

There are several options to consider. You can find another job, work part-time, or change your career. A few nurses I know have left nursing and gone into real estate, and are doing very well.

Your spouse could find a job, or a second job, until things pick up for you. If there are children, this might mean you have to stay home and care for them while your spouse goes to work. A lot of sacrifices might have to be made at this time, so be patient. Things will eventually work out.

Another option is self-employment. The trend of self-employment is rapidly becoming an option for people going through job crises. According to researchers there are about 20.5 million full-time, home-based businesses in America today.

People who work at home come in two categories: those who run their own businesses, and telecommuters employed by someone else, who work at home and commute by phone, fax, and computers.

Can you bake, sew, knit, make pottery, plant flowers, write, or do real estate? Tap into these unused gifts and talents, and use them to earn an income.

There are certain advantages to working at home. You can set your own schedule, dress the way you want, and spend more time with your family.

Build Your Job Skills

Nursing is a very competitive career, so it is very important to expand your education. If you can afford it, go back to school, get into a master's program, take special courses in computers or typing, read books, journals and magazines about nursing. In short, keep on top of your career. Even if you don't have enough money, there are scholarships available for continuing education, and community and junior colleges have courses that are quite affordable. Building up your skills gives you a better chance of finding a good job.

Conduct a Thorough Job Search

Go to a library and get books on how to write a good résumé and on how to have successful interviews. Next, look at want ads in newspapers or those posted at several hospitals. Also talk to other nurses about job offerings at the hospitals they work at.

Change Your Lifestyle

You might want to cut down on a lot of "extras" in the home. Get the family involved in this. Try preparing your own meals instead of using pre-packaged foods, or eating out. It is cheaper and healthier. Have a garage sale and sell those things you don't really need. Clip coupons, buy cheaper brands and shop for bargains. It is amazing how much you can save by cutting corners.

You might also have to put off buying new clothes; in any case, try to budget your money so as not to get into huge debts. It is very important that you continue to pay your debts and that you continue with your regular tithes. Remember, God has promised to refund you when you do. One of the blessings could be finding a job you will enjoy.

Do Something for Others

Instead of lying around doing nothing, watching TV, gossiping on the phone, or blaming others for your job woes, get busy helping others. Volunteer to work with the elderly, the disabled, or inner city kids, other disadvantaged people, homeless shelters, people with HIV and AIDS, and the needy in the local church.

Helping others will not only take your mind off your own problems, but when you see how horrific other people's problems are, this might make you count your own blessings. Keep busy and remember, "An idle mind is the devil's workshop."

Give Yourself a Treat Once in a While

Do things for yourself. Meet friends for lunch, buy yourself some flowers, take a long bubble bath, and have a positive attitude about life. Find people who will uplift you.

Let Your Church Family Know about Your Job Crisis

You need a support system at this time. Their love, concern, compassion and prayer might be just what you need. In addition, they might help support you financially, or refer you to someone who can help you and your family get back on your feet again.

Prayer: My Heavenly Father, forgive me for not putting my hope in You. Help me to trust You in this crisis I am going through right now. It is good to know that You are in control of my life, and that You know my needs even before I tell You what they are. Please help me to find a job. Right now, prepare the place You want me to be and let me not forget to say Thank You. I am grateful for all the wonderful gifts You've already given me—my family, my health, the car and the house. Most especially, thank You for sending Your only Son to die in my place. In His precious Name, I pray. Amen.

Thought: God sometimes knocks [the] prop from under us so that we'll have to trust in Him. When we don't know where the money will come from, we have no choice. We either trust in God—or sink into despair.

—Douglas Erlandson

Bibliography

Augsburger, David. *The Freedom of Forgiveness, 70 x 7*. Chicago, IL: Moody Press, 1970.

Blanchard, John. *Truth for Life*. Hertfordshire, England: Evangelical Press, 1986.

Breisch, Francis, et al. *Facing Today's Problems*. Wheaton, IL: Scripture Press Publications, 1970.

Carlson, Dwight, M.D. *Overcoming Hurts and Anger: How to Identify and Cope with Negative Emotions*. Eugene, OR: Harvest House Publishers, 1981.

Christensen, Chuck and Winnie. *Careful, Someone's Listening: Recognizing the Importance of Your Words*. Chicago, IL: Moody Press, 1990.

Conway, Jim. *Friendship: Skills for Having a Friend. . . .* Grand Rapids, MI: Zondervan Publishing House, 1989.

Davidson, Glen W. *Living with Dying*. Minneapolis, MN: Augsburg Publishing House, 1975.

Ferguson, Ben. *God, I've Got a Problem*. Ventura, CA: Vision House Publishers, 1974.

Flynn, Leslie. *The Gift of Joy*. Wheaton, IL: Victor Books, 1980.

Graham, Billy. *Angels: God's Secret Agents*. Garden City, NY: Doubleday, 1975.

Harris, Janice Long. *Secrets of People Who Love Their Work*. Downers Grove, IL: Intervarsity Press, 1992.

Hocking, David. *The Dynamic Difference*. Eugene, OR: Harvest House Publishers.

Hybels, Bill, and Mark Mittelberg. *Becoming a Contagious Christian*. Grand Rapids, MI: Zondervan Publishing House, 1994.

Kinzer, Mark. *Taming the Tongue: Why Christians Should Care about What They Say*. Ann Arbor, MI: Servant Books, 1982.

Lockerbie, Jeannette. *Salt in My Kitchen*.

Marshall, Catherine. *The Helper: He Will Meet Your Needs*. Old Tappan, NJ: Fleming H. Revell Company, 1978.

McClung, Floyd, Jr. *The Father Heart of God: God Loves You, Learn to*

Know His Compassionate Touch. Eugene, OR: Harvest House Publishers, 1985.

Miller, Patrick D. *A Little Book of Forgiveness: Challenges and Meditations for Anyone with Something to Forgive*. New York: Viking, 1994.

Minirth, Frank, M.D., et al. *The Stress Factor*. Chicago, IL: Northfield Publishing, 1992.

Neff, Miriam. *Women and their Emotions*. Chicago, IL: Moody Press, 1983.

Oates, Warren. *Managing Your Stress*. Philadelphia, PA: Fortress Press, 1985.

Remich, Ethel. *Let's Try Real Food: A Practical Guide to Nutrition and Good Health*. Grand Rapids, MI: Zondervan Publishing House, 1976.

Sherrill, Jean. *God Answers Racist Christians*. Jacksonville, AR: United We Stand Holiness Movement, 1983.

Silver, Samuel M., Rabbi. *How to Enjoy This Moment*. New York: Cornerstone Library, 1971.

Stewart, Nathaniel. *Winning Friends at Work: Your Relationships at Work Can Be More Satisfying—Personally and Professionally*. New York: Ballantine Books, 1985.

Stubblefield, Jerry. *Effective Minister of Education: A Comprehensive Handbook*. Nashville, TN: Broadman and Holman Publishers, 1993.

Sweeting, George. *Love is the Greatest*. Chicago, IL: Moody Press, 1974.

Vander Lugt, Herbert. *Light in the Valley: A Christian View of Death and Dying*. Wheaton, IL: Victor Books, 1979.

Weisinger, Hendrie, Dr., and Norman M. Lobsenz. *Nobody's Perfect: How to Give Criticism and Get Results*. Los Angeles, CA: Warner Books, 1981.

Wells, Robert G. *Prescription for Living*. San Bernardino, CA: Here's Life Publishers, Inc., 1983.

Wiersbe, Warren W. *Turning Mountains into Molehills: And Other Devotionals*. Grand Rapids, MI: Baker Book House, 1994.

Wilhelmsson, Lars. *Making Forever Friends*. Torrance, CA: Martin Press, 1982.

Wright, Norman H. *Now I Know Why I'm Depressed: And What I Can Do about It*. Eugene, OR: Harvest House Publishers, 1984.